T0392928

Craft Beers

Beer is made up of various bioactive substances containing antioxidants and specific ingredients with potentially beneficial effects on the human body if consumed in moderation. During the production process, the addition of hops, cereals, and malt leads to an increased content of naturally occurring antioxidant compounds in beer, mainly phenolic compounds. This book presents information on the history, compositional analysis, and brewing process of craft beers. It covers aspects of fruit fortification to different craft brewed beers and how it will enhance the nutritional composition, antioxidant properties, color, and sensory attributes of beers. The alcohol industry continues to grow quickly worldwide, and this book provides relevant research literature about recent studies and experimentation in beers, which will be helpful to students, researchers, industrialists, producers, and many others. The incorporation of fruits for the fortification of beers is a topic of interest, resulting in the need for more innovative and effective methods and steps in the production of newer variants of beers.

Craft Beers

Fortification, Processing, and Production

Manju Nehra
Suresh Kumar Gahlawat
Nishant Grover

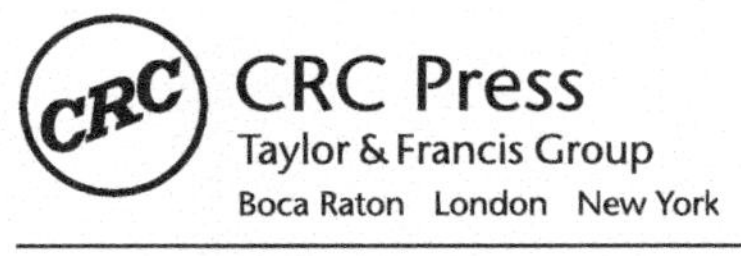

CRC Press is an imprint of the
Taylor & Francis Group, an **informa** business

Designed cover image: www.shutterstock.com/image-photo/detail-inside-mash-tun-while-making-183432398

First edition published 2023
by CRC Press
6000 Broken Sound Parkway NW, Suite 300, Boca Raton, FL 33487–2742

and by CRC Press
4 Park Square, Milton Park, Abingdon, Oxon, OX14 4RN

CRC Press is an imprint of Taylor & Francis Group, LLC

Library of Congress Cataloging-in-Publication Data
Names: Nehra, Manju, editor. | Gahlawat, Suresh Kumar, editor. | Grover, Nishant, editor.
Title: Craft beers: fortification, processing, and production / edited by Dr. Nehra Manju, Dr. S. K. Gahlawat and Nishant Grover.
Description: First edition. | Boca Raton : CRC Press, 2023. | Includes bibliographical references and index.
Identifiers: LCCN 2022044016 (print) | LCCN 2022044017 (ebook) | ISBN 9781032272573 (hardback) | ISBN 9781032272566 (paperback) | ISBN 9781003291985 (ebook)
Subjects: LCSH: Microbreweries. | Beer.
Classification: LCC TP577 .C73 2023 (print) | LCC TP577 (ebook) | DDC 663/.3—dc23/eng/20220913
LC record available at https://lccn.loc.gov/2022044016
LC ebook record available at https://lccn.loc.gov/2022044017

ISBN: 978-1-032-27257-3 (hbk)
ISBN: 978-1-032-27256-6 (pbk)
ISBN: 978-1-003-29198-5 (ebk)

DOI: 10.1201/b22906

Typeset in Times
by Apex CoVantage, LLC

Contents

Acknowledgments

Words are never enough to express gratitude towards the Almighty for blessing us with beautiful souls who were always there throughout our cynical journey. We started compiling our laboratory work for submission for the doctorate of Mr. Nishant and came up with this beautiful piece of science and art in the form of this book for readers worldwide. We are deeply overwhelmed by the support we received from the prestigious publishing house, CRC Press/Taylor & Francis. The team, including Randy and Tom, is kind and generous in always responding immediately once any queries arise.

Our heartiest thanks to our families and friends who always stood by us. The social media handles, library resources, laboratory assistance, and open-ended discussions helped us in unimaginable ways in drafting the manuscript. We sincerely thank our university authority for always being generous and helpful towards such scientific tasks. Special thanks to Honorable Vice Chancellor Professor Ajmer Singh Malik for mentoring us in the best possible ways.

We hope the readers will find the book interesting, knowledgeable, and factual.

Manju Nehra
Suresh Kumar Gahlawat
Nishant Grover

Authors

Manju Nehra heads the Food Science and Technology Department at Chaudhary Devilal University in Sirsa (Haryana, India). She has been an academic during her entire 14-year professional career. She earned her bachelor's degree in science in the medical field from Kurukshetra University in Kurukshetra, and her master's degree in science in food technology from Guru Jambheshwar University of Science and Technology in Hisar. She did her doctoral work at GJUST in Hisar. Her research focused on how natural antioxidants could prolong the shelf life of oils. She has been a Chaudhary Devilal University faculty member in Sirsa's Department of Food Science and Technology since 2007. She is actively creating new products from traditional Indian fruits, vegetables, and crops while enhancing the standard of living for farmers and rural women by educating them about simple processing and preservation methods through lectures and workshops. She has presented her findings in oral talks and posters at numerous national and international conferences. She has published more than 38 research papers in prestigious publications domestically and abroad. As the Director of Youth Welfare, she is actively helping the university's administration. She has published seven books. She connects with the public through her website so they may learn more about how human nutrition is changing. She works as a consultant for several agro-based sectors and is affiliated with several professional organizations, including AFSTI, AMI, and Punjab Science Congress. She is actively involved in both dietary counselling and curriculum development. In addition to cleanliness and nutrition, she has a keen interest in teaching, student counselling, environmental preservation, and travel.

Dr. Suresh Kumar Gahlawat is a Professor in the Department of Biotechnology at Chaudhary Devilal University in Sirsa (Haryana, India) and is currently serving as the university's Dean of Academic Affairs. He has received numerous outstanding scholarships and prizes from organizations worldwide. He is a well-known scientist who has written more than 100 research papers for reputable journals domestically and abroad. In universities in India and overseas, he has completed numerous skill-enhancement training programs and produced more than eight books. He was permitted by the Department of Biotechnology to perform advanced research at the FRS Marine Laboratory in Aberdeen, United Kingdom, from March 30, 2007 to March 7, 2008. From March 19, 2003 to March 14, 2004, he received awards from the Department of Science and Technology, the government of India in Aberdeen, the UK, and the FRS Marine Laboratory. After adopting the Integrity Pledge to keep the highest standards of honesty and integrity and to follow goodness and the rule of law in all aspects of life, he was given a Certificate of Commitment by the Central Vigilance Commission, Satarkta Bhawan, GPO Complex, INA, New Delhi. He has visited a variety of labs, including the University of Stirling in the UK, the Marine Laboratory in Aberdeen, the FRS BBSRC in Pirbright, the reference lab for IPN and SVC viruses, and the CEFAS in Weymouth, UK (working on DNA vaccines and real-time PCR). Several gene sequences/SNPs have been submitted to GenBank,

NCBI (USA), by Professor Gahlawat. He has guided many PhD scholars and MSc students and mentored hundreds of learners to pursue their careers in academics and industries. He has served as chairperson of various departments in the university and held different administrative positions including Dean of Student Welfare, Dean of Colleges, Dean of Faculty, and Dean of Research. He contributes to the science fraternity by motivating young scientists with his enthusiastic approach. He has completed four R&D projects from UGC, ICAR, and the government of Haryana. His research interests include the development of molecular diagnostic methods for bacterial and viral diseases.

Nishant Grover is an emerging scientist, and, under the direction of Dr. Manju Nehra, he is working on his PhD in the Food Science and Technology Department. He has experience working as a consultant for many craft breweries and is currently working on improvising brews using various fruit sources. He has participated in multiple workshops and conferences related to food science. He is actively involved in product development from various indigenous food sources and has published research articles in journals of national and international repute.

Conflict of Interest

The authors state that there is no potential bias in their work. Nobody other than the authors of the study participated in the process of designing the study, producing the manuscript, or deciding whether or not to publish the results. In addition, the information, data, and research that were reprinted in the preparation of the manuscript are appropriately recognized in the bibliography/references. There are citations for each table and image, indicating where the information was originally gathered. There is not the slightest intention of plagiarizing any of the content cited in the sources. The majority of the data is from the laboratory of the authors. If the writers are located, they will be held accountable for the act. (The publisher will not be considered responsible for any act of plagiarism or data copying.) Following a thorough review by the program Grammarly, the document was found to contain less than 10% duplicate content across all of the chapters.

Dr. Manju Nehra
Chairperson
Food Science and Technology
Chaudhary Devilal University, Sirsa

1 Brewing and Malting

1.1 INTRODUCTION

The most consumed and widely known alcoholic beverage worldwide is beer, which is also one of the oldest. Since the beginning of civilization, humans have engaged in activities such as making and drinking beer. Before the invention of bread, the original beer mainly was manufactured from grain, water, and spontaneous fermentation caused by wild airborne yeast (Campbell, 2017). Around 5000 BCE, the Egyptians are said to have been the first to record the making of beer; nevertheless, it is also thought that the earliest known brewers were from archaic Mesopotamian societies. In the early Middle Ages, German monks introduced hop as a bittering and flavoring ingredient, giving rise to modern beer. A considerably larger scale of beer manufacturing was made possible by the Industrial Revolution, which saw a shift in beer production from the household to mass production (Aroh, 2019).

Commercial brewing of beer involves the carefully regulated fermentation of wort, a liquid made from malted barley that is high in sugars, nitrogenous chemicals, sulphur compounds, and trace elements. The chemical expression for fermentation, which turns glucose into ethanol and carbon dioxide, is:

$$C_6H_{12}O_6 + 2Pi + 2ADP \rightarrow 2C_2H_5OH + 2CO_2 + 2ATP$$

Beer is brewed by the controlled fermentation of brewer's wort, a barley juice extracted from malted barley high in sugars, nitrogenous chemicals, sulfur compounds, and trace components. Fermentation is the process by which glucose is converted into ethanol and carbon dioxide.

There is a series of complex biochemical reactions under this chemical reaction. Numerous enzymes are used in these processes, also referred to as the "Embden-Meyerhof-Parnas route" or the "glycolytic pathway," which take place anaerobically inside the cells of brewing yeast (Campbell, 2017). Beer fermentation is a continuous process that takes five to seven days to complete. After the ethanol has formed, the beer is transferred to maturation vessels, and the flavor is naturally refined. Following this, the product is developed into a variety of different brands (Campbell, 2017). Microbial activity is present throughout the whole brewing process from the raw materials production and malting. While most of these actions are positive, some pose risks to the ultimate product's quality and must be actively regulated through careful management (Bokulich & Bamforth, 2013).

DOI: 10.1201/b22906-1

1.2 BEER

Beer is an alcoholic beverage produced by brewing and fermenting grains, often malted barley hops, and then flavored with other ingredients to make it a little bitter. With moderate consumption, beer is considered to provide a number of health advantages. A few of these fascinating health advantages include anti-cancer properties; lowered risk of cardiovascular diseases; increased bone density; prevention of diabetes, anemia, and hypertension; anti-aging properties; prevention of gallstones, dementia, and coronary disease; aiding digestion, kidney stones, and osteoporosis; stress relief; and acting as a diuretic (Ore et al., 2018).

There are many other kinds of microorganisms used to make beer, including lactic bacteria and yeast, but *Saccharomyces cerevisiae* (brewer's yeast) is typically employed since it is widely available at a reasonable price. The handling of grains, malting or germination, mashing or extraction with water, filtering, and fermentation are the main steps in the production of beer. Once the necessary malt quality has been reached, the germination process is stopped; green brown malt is transformed into a stable, storable product; color and taste are also developed; enzymes are stabilized and conserved; and undesirable flavors are eliminated. The goals of mashing include the extraction and hydrolysis of starch, sugars, proteins, and non-starch polysaccharides; solubilization and dissolving of grain components; and establishment of a fermentable sugar profile. The fermentation process establishes the alcohol content, taste character, and carbonation level of the beer. After completion of fermentation, yeast flocculates, and that makes easy to separate it from beer. Temperatures during cold maturation will affect beer clarity (Ore et al., 2018).

Beer has been brewed since ancient times and is being enjoyed today with only few modifications to the recipe. The primary component is malted barley, which, after being milled and mashed (heated with water) to extract its nutrients, yields wort, a nutritious mixture rich in protein and sugar (known as brewer's wort). It is the perfect medium for yeast to grow and ferment. Hops are added during the boiling of wort since it was discovered that hops possess anti-bacterial characteristics that conserve the wort and preserve fermented beer, giving the beer a pleasantly bitter taste (Campbell, 2017).

For many years, a slow-batch fermentation procedure carried out in a single fermentation vessel was the only way of fermenting beer that was known to exist. This approach had drawbacks in terms of quality and cost. Due to the long fermentation time, several tanks were needed to accommodate all of the beer batches that were in the fermentation process, resulting in the high costs of vessels and the associated costs of holding these vessels at the required temperatures and testing the quality of each batch. Furthermore, there was no assurance that the flavor of the beer would remain constant. Recent times have seen the introduction of continuous fermentation, which includes recycling some of the fermented beer back to the wort at the beginning of the fermentation process. The ultimate result is a continual flow of beer. In a continuous system, the wort brewing stage may be completed at a time suitable for the brewery. The boiled wort is chilled to 0°C (the wort does not freeze at this temperature because of its high sugar content) and held in storage tanks where protein material (which would otherwise make the beer appear cloudy or "hazy") precipitates out. Continuous fermentation uses this system of cold wort storage. Up until the point when it must be continuously delivered to the fermentation, the wort is kept in the storage vessel. For several days, one wort storage tank will continually flow into the fermentation (Campbell, 2017).

The yeast strain used, along with the composition of the wort, affects the flavor and fragrance of any beer in a significant way. Additionally, the efficacy of the fermentation process is significantly influenced by yeast characteristics, including flocculation and fermentation capacity (including the absorption of wort sugars, amino acids, short peptides, and ammonium ions), osmotic pressure, ethanol tolerance, and oxygen needs. Individual brewers' proprietary strains are often fiercely guarded and preserved (Stewart, 2016). Numerous varietal strains of yeast have been developed by genetic modification, and this, along with adjustments to the brewing process, has produced a variety of beers.

Beer, like any fermented food, is a microbial product. Microbial activity is involved in every step of its production, defining the many characteristics that contribute to final quality. While fermentation of cereal extracts by *Saccharomyces* is the most important microbial process involved in brewing, a vast array of other microbes affects the complete process (Bokulich & Bamforth, 2013). The diagram that follows shows an overview of bacterial and fungal species previously reported at all major stages of beer production.

The beers that are most frequently seen are:

Lager: Beers brewed with yeast (*Saccharomyces carlsbergensis*) that sinks to the bottom of the vessel. As a consequence, all the yeast and other debris sink to the bottom, producing clear beer.

The colorless lager beer that was first made in the city of Pilsen is known as pilsner. Compared to lager water, the water used for this variety of beer tends to be harder and contains more calcium and magnesium. Pilsner beer has a paler hue than lager beer does.

Ale: Beers brewed with yeast (*Saccharomyces cerevisiae*) that floats to the top of the fermentation tanks, producing cloudier beer. They often contain more alcohol than lagers.

A particularly black ale is called a porter. By toasting the malt before brewing, richer colors and distinctive flavors are produced. Typically, this has a stronger taste and contains more alcohol.

An extremely dark beer that is nearly black is stout. The roasted malt or barley is what gives the beer its dark color and roasted flavor (Wong, 2003).

1.3 BREWING: BEER PRODUCTION

Brewing is a massively complicated process that uses yeast to primarily turn water, malt, and hops into what we know as beer. The wide range of beers is mostly a result of the various production-stage conditions (temperature, kind of grain, etc.)

(Sánchez, 2017). Malt can be partially replaced with additives rich in starch, such as rice, corn, or wheat. The malt enzymes, mostly amylases but also proteases, break down starch and proteins when a mixture of barley malt and brewing water (referred to as "mash") is boiled to a temperature of around 60°C, producing a mixture of carbohydrates and peptides or amino acids. For that reason, barley has to go through a regulated germination process so that these enzymes can develop in the grain before mashing. Barley malt is the name of this germinated barley (De Keukeleire, 2000).

Heating halts the conversion of starch to sugar. Pale, amber, and even black malts can be produced, depending on the circumstances (temperature, time), with the color coming from the caramelization of sugars. It's vital to note that the color of the malt(s) used determines the color of the finished beer. Furthermore, it is clear that colored malts have a unique flavor, which is frequently a hallmark of certain dark brews. After filtering, the sugar solution, or "wort," as it is known in the brewing industry, is transferred to the brewing kettle and cooked for at least an hour while hops (*Humulus lupulus* L.) are being added. In comparison to the huge amounts of malt utilized in the brewing, far fewer hops are required. Hops also sterilize the wort solution in addition to creating insoluble complexes with proteins and polypeptides (which help keep beer stable). The bitter flavor that hops impart to beers, especially blond ones, is their most valuable feature. Additionally, hops are essential for the stability of beer froth (De Keukeleire, 2000).

After cooling and the removal of spent hops, the liquid known as "hopped wort" is pumped to the fermentation vessels, and yeast is added under aeration for growth. During the anaerobic phase, yeast cells convert sugars to ethanol and carbon dioxide. Depending on the temperature during fermentation and the nature of yeast collection at the end of the fermentation period, beers are distinguished as being produced by "bottom fermentation" or "top fermentation." Yeast strains, appropriate for bottom-fermented beers (*Saccharomyces carlsbergensis*), are active below 5°C, and they settle to the bottom of the fermenter after production of about 5% ethanol. Conversely, yeasts typical for the production of top-fermented beers (*Saccharomyces cerevisiae*) operate at ambient temperature and resist higher concentrations of ethanol up to 12%. When the activity stops, the yeast cells collect at the top as a dense foam (De Keukeleire, 2000).

A typical fermentation lasts approximately a week, producing what is known as "green beer" or "young beer," which is unpalatable due to the formation of a variety of offensive (poor taste and smell) chemicals. Therefore, beers require a maturation or lagering period of several weeks at roughly 0°C, during which the undesirable components are gradually broken down. Beer cannot be packed until the content has fallen below critical levels. Beers may undergo pasteurisation for extended preservation. Specialty beers frequently require a slow second fermentation (over several months), typically in oak kegs, to produce sour flavors (De Keukeleire, 2000).

1.3.1 Malting

The best cereal grain for brewing and malting is barley. It has a husk to shield the germ, a high starch-to-protein ratio for high yields, a full enzyme system, a self-adjusting pH, and light color, making it self-contained. Wheat and rye are also frequently malted for brewing in addition to barley. Although buckwheat and spelt may also be malted, the resulting malt does not function as effectively in the brewhouse as malted barley.

The fundamental malting procedure still consists of three steps—steeping, germination, and drying—although it's more of an exact science now than when man first dipped baskets of grain into open wells in Mesopotamia 5,000 years ago to prepare it for brewing.

Barley is modified to malt, which is also known as processed barley. Malt can be divided into two primary groups: base malts and speciality malts. Base malts have high concentrations of the enzymes, complex carbohydrates, and sugars required for fermentation. When the duration, temperature, or humidity of the three steps of the malting process—steeping, germination, and drying—are changed to create individual tastes and colors or particular functions, specialty malts are created. In order to contribute distinctive flavors like intense malt, sweet caramel, nutty, woody, coffee, or burned, as well as rich colors ranging from golden to red to black, many specialty malts are made to be used in smaller amounts. This is because more intense heating reduces the amount of enzymes available for fermentation. Production of specialty malts differs from basic malting in that batch sizes are typically smaller, it requires significantly more labor and resources and more laboratory testing for consistency, and it calls for constant attention from an experienced maltster who relies on his senses of sight, taste, smell, and touch to produce the desired finished product from start to finish.

1.3.2 Steeping

The first step of malting is steeping, in which barley is soaked in water. During steeping, water is absorbed by the raw barley kernel, and germination begins. Steeping starts with raw barley that has been sorted and cleaned, then transferred into deep tanks and covered with water. For the next 40 to 48 hours, the raw barley alternates between submerged and drained until it increases in moisture content from about 12% to about 44%.

The absorbed water activates naturally existing enzymes and stimulates the embryo to develop new enzymes. The enzymes break down the protein and carbohydrate matrix that encloses starch granules in the endosperm, opening up the seed's starch reserves, and newly developed hormones initiate growth of the acrospire (sprout).

Steeping is complete when the barley has reached a sufficient moisture level to allow uniform breakdown of the starches and proteins. One visual indicator that the maltster uses to determine the completion of steeping is to count the percentage of kernels that show "chit." Raw barley that has been properly steeped is referred to as "chitted" barley," the "chit" being the start of the rootlets that are now visibly emerging from the embryo of the kernel (Kunze, 2004).

1.3.3 Germination

The chitted barley is moved from the tank to the germination compartment using a procedure known as "steep out." In the germination tank, the barley modifies to malt while germination starts in the steeping tank.

The term "modification" describes the breakdown of the protein and carbs, which causes the starch reserves in the seeds to become accessible. The barley has to stay in the compartment for four or five days for a good alteration. By forcing humidified air that has been temperature-adjusted through the bed, germination may be regulated. Turners prevent the bed from felting and clumping together as a result of rootlet growth.

1.3.4 Drying (Kilning)

Germination is stopped by drying (kilning). If germination isn't stopped, the kernel will keep expanding, and develops into a plant that would consume all the starch reserves required by the brewer. Base malts are generally dried for two to four hours at a temperature of 180–190°F. This produces tastes that range from being quite light to being subtly malty, whereas specialty malts may be roasted, dried at higher temperatures for extended periods of time, or both. Each unique malt's flavor and color traits are developed by varying the moisture content, drying time, and temperature (Kunze, 2004).

1.3.5 Brewing Steps

1.3.5.1 Milling

Malt kernels are physically crushed during milling mashing, which is done immediately prior to use in mashing. To achieve a grind that is neither too fine nor too coarse, the different milling operations must be properly adjusted. If milling is finer, more sweet wort can be extracted, but it will form more clumps and get sticky.

Also, husk is desired as it works as a filter bed during lautering. In order for the sparge water to properly rinse the sugars out of the mash, pulverized husk cannot be used to "fluff up" the grain bed. On the other hand, a very coarse grind would minimize the surface area of the grist that is exposed to the grain enzymes, even though it would result in a well-draining grain bed in the lauter tun. Thus, there may not be adequate conversion of β-glucan, protein, and starch.

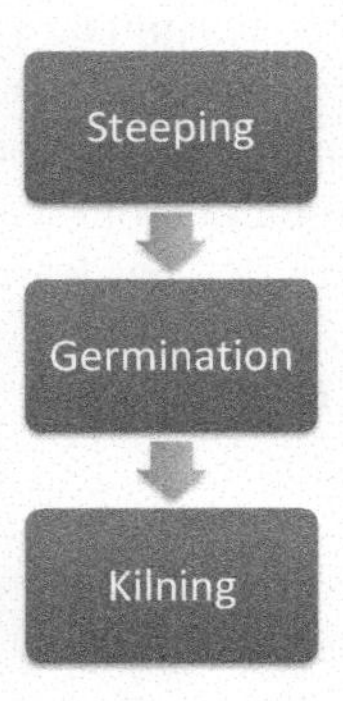

FIGURE 1.1 Malting Process

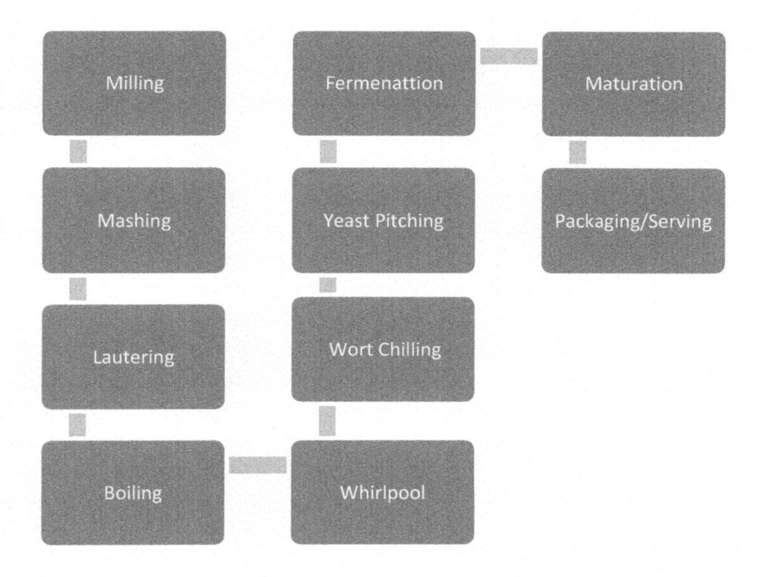

FIGURE 1.2 Hop Structure

Usually, coarse milling is done (70% coarse, 30% fine) except in the case of mash filters. Usually, two roller mills are used in microbreweries, and six roller mills are used in commercial ones. The actual grind that is employed by the majority of brewers in the real world is a balance between theory and reality since both overly fine and excessively coarse grinds result in a decrease in brewhouse extract yield. Therefore, the mill must be set to produce a mealy rather than chunky or floury grist for the best brewhouse efficiency and yield. The gap setting depends on a variety of variables, including the type, size, hardness, and friability of the kernels; the method used to prepare the grist for milling (wet or dry); and the type of machinery used to mill the grain.

In order to prevent a poor runoff or blocked mash, a combined mash-lauter tun (such as is used for single-temperature infusion mashes in the UK and in certain small breweries worldwide) often requires a rather coarse grind. A mash filter can handle an almost flour-like grind, but a separate lauter tun can often handle a finer grind for higher extract efficiency. Thus, a mash filter is by far the most effective wort-extraction tool available. However, it is also the most costly; thus, it is often only used in larger breweries (Eaton, 2017).

1.3.6 Mashing

Milled grains are mixed with water to create the "mash," which resembles porridge; the process is referred to as mashing. The sweet fermentable liquid known as the wort is created by the conversion of malt and other cereal starches into sugars and the solubilization of proteins and other substances in the mash. Whole kernels of malt are brought into the brewery from the malting plant, where they are subsequently ground to create the grain combination known as "grist." The mash is created by combining the grain with precisely measured amounts of warm or hot water. The temperature profile of mash varies depending on the beer style and the grains used. Usually, grist ratio (water-malt ratio) for mashing is 2.7:1 to 3:1.

Infusion mashing, decoction mashing, and temperature-controlled infusion mashing are the three fundamental types of mashing processes. Depending on local custom, the type of malt available, the tools being used, and the types of beers being brewed, different mashing techniques are employed across the world.

Specially grown barley types are used to make malts. At the time of malting, enzymes begin to degrade the "starchy endosperm," the bulk of the kernel. A framework of cell walls, primarily hemicelluloses, which is full of starch granules bound in a protein matrix, makes up the starchy endosperm. During malting and mashing, proteins, hemicelluloses, and starch are divided into smaller, soluble fractions, which are then washed off during sparging to create wort. A mashing procedure is used to release as much soluble material into the wort as possible while avoiding unfavorable components, depending on malting technique.

The mashing tank is equipped with an agitator that ensures uniform mixing of mash and helps in proper starch breakdown. Mashing usually takes one to two hours, depending on the beer style and mashing regime.

The various mashing profiles are used to extract as much soluble material as possible from various malts. Different temperatures are applied to the mash throughout the mashing process, which is good for breaking down the various components of the starchy endosperm. Proteases degrade the protein matrix binding the starch granules within a temperature range of 35 to 45°C (95 to 113°F). Amylases break down the starch granules and function best at 61 to 67°C (141.8 to 152.6°F), whereas glucanases break down the hemicellulose gums and have an optimal temperature range of 45 to 55°C (113 to 131°F).

The majority of ales were historically brewed using an infusion mashing technique. To do this, high-quality, well-modified malt is mashed into a "mash tun" and kept there for at least an hour at a temperature of 65°C (149°F). During this time, the enzymes in the malt function to release the malt sugars and other components from the grain. The wort—the sweet liquid that the yeast will ferment into beer—is made of all the soluble components that make up the mash. This wort is then sprayed with hot water, known as sparging (at roughly 75°C), which passes through the mash and out of the mash tun through a slotted false bottom. Because just one temperature is employed, this infusion procedure is also referred to as isothermal infusion mashing. Many craft brewers employ infusion mashing to create lagers, wheat beers, and other types of beers as the quality of malting barley rises. The infusion mashing technique is still popular among small brewers and pub breweries since it only needs two brewhouse containers (a mash/lauter vessel and a kettle) to generate hopped wort.

The majority of lager and some ales are brewed using a technique called temperature-programmed infusion mashing. In this method, an infusion mash is heated through a sequence of temperature increases, rested at each temperature for a certain amount of time, and then heated through the next series of temperature increases.

Sometimes, these temperature rest are referred to as "stands." By feeding steam or hot water through heating panels built into the mashing vessel's walls, which are also equipped with an agitator to guarantee proper mixing, the mash is heated. In a mashing vessel, also known as a conversion vessel, the malt is typically mashed at around 45 to 50°C (113 to 122°F) to begin. In order to let enzymes operate on the protein and gums in the grist and liberate the starch from which the malt sugars are generated, the mash is frequently kept at this temperature for anywhere between 10 and 25 minutes. To create amino acids, which are essential for the growth of yeast during fermentation, the proteins must be broken down. In order to prevent them from subsequently contributing to unwelcome haze in the final beer, higher weight protein components are also broken down. Other proteinaceous materials can contribute to beer foam, and a prolonged protein rest or stand at 45°C (113°F) can harm a beer's ability to froth. The mash is heated to 62–67°C (143.6–152.6°F) for the saccharification stand after the protein rest. These temperatures are ideal for the amylase enzymes, which convert starch and larger sugar molecules into fermentable sugars. The amount of grain used has a significant impact on how much sugar is generated in the mash. However, differing saccharification temperatures will result in various wort sugars and thus various beers. Low saccharification temperature mashes result in a higher proportion of fermentable sugars in the wort, which results in a drier beer with a higher alcohol level. In contrast, saccharification temperatures at the top of the range will lead to fewer fermentable worts and sweeter, fuller-bodied beers; these will be produced from the same amount of grain and have a lower alcohol level. The mash must be heated to a final temperature of around 75°C (167°F) before being transferred to a device for mash separation, often a lauter tun. This last temperature increase renders the enzymes inactive and lowers the viscosity of the wort, resulting in a speedier outflow. "Mashing off" is a common term used to describe this. The ideal way to make some varieties of beer is to use infusion mashes that have been precisely designed and temperature programmed to carry out specific tasks. For instance, a lot of wheat-based beers are mashed with longer protein rests (wheat contains more protein than malting barley) or other rests that are intended to encourage the formation of particular characteristics in the finished beer. Therefore, the brewer may precisely adjust the wort to get the desired flavor (Eaton, 2017).

The term "decoction mashing" refers to an earlier temperature-programmed mashing procedure employed by conventional continental brewers, frequently for the brewing of lager. Before temperature-programmed infusion mashing equipment was established, decoction mashing was employed, and European malts were frequently undermodified at that time. Part of a mash is decocted by transferring it from a mash vessel into a mash cooker, where it is heated to 100°C (212°F) and quickly boiled. The original mash vessel, which has been warmed throughout the mixing process, receives the boiling mash after a certain amount of time. For instance, mash at 45°C (113°F) may be removed from a mash vessel, cooked, and then put back in the mash vessel. The blended mash temperature will increase to the desired saccharification temperature of 65°C (149°F) while the mash vessel is swirled. This procedure can be repeated many times, enabling the mash to reach a variety of temperature stands. A "single," "double," or even "triple" decoction procedure may be used in decoction mashing; the latter is now very uncommon. With today's malts and brewing equipment, decoction mashing isn't absolutely essential anymore, although some brewers still think it adds depth to the malt taste. Many others are doubtful and believe the approach is unduly energy and labor intensive.

When unmalted grains, often corn grits or rice, are added as adjuncts to the mash, variations on decoction techniques are sometimes utilized. The unmalted grain is combined with hot water in a different container, commonly referred to as a "rice cooker" or "grits cooker," and this mash is cooked to 100°C (212°F). A tiny amount of malted barley is then added. At this temperature, the hard starches in uncooked grains gelatinize, making them pliable and amenable to enzyme breakdown. The enzymes in the barley malt mash will convert the now-gelatinized cereal starches into sugars when this "cereal mash" is introduced. This method is used to make light-bodied, light-flavored lager beers all over the world, and it is almost always employed to brew mass-market beers in the United States.

1.3.7 Lautering

A fluid combination of dissolved and undissolved ingredients remains after the mashing process. The insoluble portion of the extract is known as the spent grains, while the aqueous solution is known as brewer's wort. Only the wort is utilized for making beer; thus, it must be separated as fully as possible from the spent grains. The spent grains are mostly made up of the husk, the seedling, and other materials that do not dissolve during mashing or have precipitated again during wort collection. Mashing is followed by lautering, in which the wort is separated from the grains. The extract should be recovered as much as possible throughout the lautering process. In the filtration process known as lautering, the spent grains serve as the filter material.

This sweet liquid or wort is mixture of sugars in which some are fermentable while others are not; this provides richness to finished beer. Wort passes through the sieve of false bottom of the lauter tank; grains stay above that. It usually takes between 90 minutes and 2 hours. After lautering, the grain bed left, which is known as spent grain, is collected for cattle feed.

There are two distinct phases that follow: running off the first wort (primary mash) and sparging (washing out) the spent grains (second wort).

The first wort is the liquid that drains from the used grains. The spent grains still contain extract after the wort has been removed. Recovery of this extract is required for efficient functioning, so, when the initial wort has runoff, the spent grains are sparged. The wort is gradually diluted by sparging.

The first wort must include 4–6% more extract than the intended beer: for example, for a 12 °Plato (°P) beer, it must contain 16 to 18% in order to achieve the correct wort concentration at the conclusion of lautering.

Hot water is used to remove the extract that the spent grains retained. This action is referred to as sparging. The second wort that runs off is the thinner substance. Its extract content gradually diminishes over time because only a small amount of the final extract can be successfully removed from the spent grains; this is mostly a diffusion process (Kunze, 2004).

The amount of water needed for sparging is determined by the quantity and concentration of the initial wort as well as the concentration that has to be attained in the kettle. The discarded grains are extracted more thoroughly and, as a result, provide a better yield when more sparging water is poured through them. However, the more water that must be evaporated again, the more water that is passed through the used grains. Therefore, a balance between lautering time and yield and boiling time and energy expenditures must be established (Eaton, 2017).

More sparging water may be utilized the more concentrated the first wort is since a higher concentration necessarily results in a lower volume of first wort. Therefore, a larger yield is likewise attained with a higher first wort percentage. Thus, the lautering temperature is crucial.

Filtration happens more quickly when the temperature rises because the viscosity of the liquid drops. Accordingly, lautering would occur most quickly at 100°C. While residual undissolved starch is always removed from the spent grains during sparging, late saccharification by α-amylase can only take place if the enzyme has not been rendered inactive by temperatures higher than about 78°C. Therefore, lautering at 100°C always yields blue mashes. In this instance, adding malt extract to the fermentation cellar is an attempt to make up for the error; however, it has unfavorable effects. Because β-amylase is quickly degraded above 78°C, lautering must be done at a lower temperature.

More or less bright is the wort that is pouring off. In the lauter tun, the level of turbidity is particularly susceptible to change. Fatty acids and breakdown products are present in the compounds that cause haze, and yeast needs them for the synthesis of new cell components. Therefore, turbid worts frequently result in a fermentation period of one or two days. Additionally, tests have demonstrated that beers made from wort with a turbidity of 40 EBC taste a little bit fresher, richer, more palatable, more flowery, purer, softer, and more enjoyable with a cleaner bitter flavor, and they generally have more character. These brews, however, do not age as well as other types of beer. Therefore, lautering is advised with a setting of 20 EBC turbidity value and no cold break removal.

Sparging is carried out in the hop kettle until the necessary concentration is attained. The term "last runnings" refers to the low proportion of wort that runs off last. The last runnings of a standard beer (Vollbier) still contain roughly 2–3% of extract; lengthier sparging is uneconomical since the expenses of evaporating the additional amount of sparging water would far outweigh the advantages of greater extract (cost-benefit threshold). For the subsequent brew, this is occasionally utilized as mashing-in water or sparging water. In the case of Bockbier, the spent grains cannot be sufficiently sparged since doing so would result in an excessive reduction in wort concentration. The leftover worts from these beers are frequently utilized as mashing-in water for lighter beer (Einfachbier), which is brewed as the next batch.

As the sparging process comes to a close, larger volumes of unwanted material enter solution. Long-chained fatty acids in particular have a considerable influence, especially with regard to the flavor stability of the beer, together with mineral matter such as silicic acid (SiO_2) and polyphenols. It was demonstrated that in comparable experiments on a turbid (140 EBC) and clear (16 EBC) wort, the fraction of long-chained fatty acids and oxidized lipid oxidation products, such as hexanal, pentanal, and nonalactone, increase disproportionately in the turbid wort. The beer's flavor and flavor stability suffer as a result. It is advised to treat the final 10% of the second-to-last batch of wort with activated carbon (3 g/hl) in order to avoid this. After returning it, the treatment for both is continued until 10 minutes remain in the boiling time. Tests reveal that beer handled in this manner has significantly increased flavor stability.

In this context, it's important to give careful consideration to using the previous batches of beer as mash-in liquor. Long-term sparging and recycling of previous runs increase production but lower quality. Therefore, the wort quality should be taken into account in relation to the extract yield.

However, if the leftovers must be utilized, then they should be treated with active carbon to get rid of any unwanted flavorings. Therefore, the last wort is frequently used to finish sparging.

The term "economic threshold for use of last runnings" refers to the restrictions that the increased energy costs impose in addition to quality concerns about the use of untreated last runnings. The use of final runnings is profitable only when the value of the extra extract is greater than the price of the energy necessary to evaporate the water. As a result, the threshold for using final runnings is influenced by the nation's energy and malt prices.

A lauter tun or a mash filter is used to separate the mash.

1.3.7.1 Spent Grains

On spent grain discharge, around 100–130 kg of spent grains—or 21–22 kg of spent grains per hl of beer—are produced from 100 kg of malt and include 70–80% water. Dried spent grains are composed of approximately 28% protein, 8.2% fat, 41% nitrogen-free extract, 17.5% cellulose, and 5.3 % inorganic material. If feasible, the spent grains are sold as animal feed. The same amount of discarded grain has around one-fifth the nutritional content of equal amounts of barley. This is logical if you keep in mind that the maximum amount of extract is extracted while mashing. The benefit of wasted grain is that it digests more easily than the original grain.

The spent grains lacks vitamins so they can't be used as animal feed but somehow due to cost effectiveness and easy availability farmers use spent grains as animal feed.

However, there isn't always or everywhere a need for spent grains at nearby farms. In that scenario, they must be quickly and satisfactorily disposed of before they spoil and begin to smell.

However, it is becoming more challenging for brewers to eliminate discarded grains. Therefore, more and more brewers are beginning to dry and burn the used grains. This allows for the recovery of a sizeable portion of the energy consumed in the brewhouse. Another method involves fermenting the used grains to create biogas, which may then be burned to recover energy.

1.3.8 Boiling

After that, wort is transferred to the boiling kettle and boiled for 60 to 90 minutes. Hops are added to the kettle at the start of boiling for bitterness and at the end for aroma and flavor; α-acids, present in hops, convert to iso-α-acids. These iso-α-acids are responsible for the unique bitterness of beers.

The extraction and transformation of hop components, the formation and precipitation of protein-polyphenol compounds, the sterilization of the wort, the destruction of all enzymes, the thermal exposure of the wort, the lowering of the pH of the wort, the formation of reducing substances, and the evaporation of unfavorable aroma components all take place during the wort boiling process.

Boiling also causes some water to evaporate, concentrating the wort and somewhat intensifying the color.

Proteins precipitate concurrently with the transport of bitter and aromatic hop components into the wort during boiling.

1.3.9 Wort Sterilization

Numerous bacteria and molds that, if left unchecked, can quickly turn beer sour or alter its flavor enter the mash with the malt dust. The wort is sterilized, and all the microorganisms included in the wort are eliminated during the boiling process.

1.3.10 Isomerization of Hops

Hop resins, often known as bitter compounds, are the most crucial part of hops for making beer since they give the beverage its bitter flavor. Other significant hop components include hop oil and hop polyphenols.

In cold wort, the α-acid are fully insoluble. Isomerization, or modifications to the α-acid structure, take place in boiling wort. Compared to the α-acid from which they are derived, the iso-compounds that are created are far more soluble.

While boiling, α-acid is not entirely isomerized. Only approximately one-third of the additional α-acid is typically recovered as iso-compounds in the boiling wort. Furthermore, significant amounts of bitter substances are eliminated throughout the succeeding stages of beer manufacturing.

Isohumulone: Various α-acid components isomerized to varying degrees determine the isohumulone yield on boiling and, as a result, the bitterness of the beer. The best isohumulone yield is provided by cohumulone. A bitterer beer may be made by utilizing hop varietals with a greater percentage of cohumulone, such as Northern Brewer.

Boiling time: The production of isohumulone rises with longer boiling times. At the start of boiling, most of the α-acid is isomerized, and as boiling proceeds, the isomerization rate gradually declines. The majority of the bittering agents are isomerized after one hour of boiling.

The pH: A higher pH always promotes greater isomerization, while lower pH always produces bitterness that is thought to be more harmonious and refined.

The isohumulone production falls when more hops are added, which affects the humulone concentration. However, the reduction only applies to a small range (up to 10%). During the break, a substantial portion of the isohumulone is absorbed. Increasing isomerization, for instance, using hotter temperatures

Size of the extracted hop fragments: Milling hops speeds up the extraction process and enhance bitter substances' output.

The more time wort is boiled, the more volatile hop oil becomes. The intensity and pleasantness of the aromas produced by various hop oils vary more widely. Therefore, keeping some of the finest hop oil in the wort and the beer is preferred. To preserve at least some of the greatest hop oil, the aroma hops, which have the best fragrances, are often introduced just 15 to 20 minutes before casting in most breweries, provided this is given value. The last hops can be added while the whirlpool is running, although this could cause trub issues.

Hop polyphenols readily dissolve in water: The anthocyanogens, tannins, and catechins are all types of hop polyphenols. They are crucial to the break formation process.

The anti-oxidizing properties of the polyphenols have a favorable impact on the beer's flavor stability. Thus, the polyphenol's oxidation resistance acts as a complement to the sulphite's oxidation resistance. Therefore, when mashing, one should strive for a higher polyphenol content while avoiding oxygen at all costs.

1.3.11 Protein Precipitation

The high-molecular-weight proteins, to the extent that they are soluble, have a tendency to coagulate when heated due to their large molecule size. They achieve this by forming a link with the hop and malt polyphenols, hastening the coagulation.

As a result, the malt's polyphenols respond more slowly than those in hops. Since the proteins have variable molecular sizes and the polyphenols are partially oxidized, a wide range of molecules with diverse behaviors are produced:

> When heated, proteins, polyphenols, nitrogen-containing chemicals, and oxidised polyphenols become insoluble and precipitate as break during wort boiling. Break refers to the observable break flakes that occur during wort boiling. A coarse flaking break was usually an indication of effective protein precipitation and effective stability against haze formation. In the past, precipitating these chemicals was always thought to be beneficial. This needed a lengthy boiling time, which was always 2 hours up to a recent time.
>
> (Hough et al., 1982)

Energy costs have been rising steadily in the interim, and techniques for removing haze-causing elements from beer have been developed. Since not all coagulable protein must be precipitated, a portion should be kept for improved foam retention; protein precipitation is now seen from a new perspective.

Modern wort-boiling techniques prevent prolonged, vigorous boiling in order to achieve this. As a result, high-molecular-weight proteins that would ordinarily precipitate during prolonged and intense boiling remain dissolved in the wort, raising the possibility of improved foam retention. Furthermore, a quicker and less intense boiling process results in lower energy expenses.

The (clear) finished wort has a total nitrogen content of about 1,000 mg/L. About 200 mg/L (150–350 Mg/L) of this can precipitate nitrogen when combined with magnesium sulfate ($MgSO_4$-N). High-molecular-weight protein components are found using this technique. The beer foam and $MgSO_4$-N are closely related to one another. A better foam retention is predicted by a higher $MgSO_4$-N value. Additionally, the free amino nitrogen (FAN), which is used to identify the amino acids and final amino groups of peptides and proteins, is assessed in the completed wort. The pitching wort must have 220–250 mg of free amino nitrogen/l to ensure a successful fermentation; 100 to 120 mg/L FAN still remain in the beer since the yeast cannot use all the amino acids.

More coagulable nitrogen stays in the wort, increasing the likelihood of greater foam retention, thanks to shorter boiling times, gentler boiling at lower temperatures, and less shear pressure. The ideal level of coagulable nitrogen in cold wort is 20–40 mg/L. Additionally, there is a decrease in the creation of chemicals that are related to ageing.

However, enough evaporation of free DMS (100 Mg/L) must be paid attention to. Additionally, improved fermentation as a result of biological wort acidification results in greater foam properties.

1.3.12 Evaporation

Water evaporates as a result of a prolonged boiling process. This has traditionally been given a lot of weight since it was believed that good protein precipitation (break formation) could be achieved by the strong movement of the kettle's contents.

Only a few decades ago, a high rate of condensation was a requirement for a wort kettle's AAR, and a kettle with a rate of wort evaporation of 10–15% was regarded as a high-performance tie. This has altered since then, as evidenced. Today, a rate of evaporation of 4% is desired with excellent evaporation efficiency.

The amount of water that evaporates during the boiling process is used to calculate evaporation (total evaporation). The total evaporation displays the amount of unboiled wort that has been evaporated overall.

Water evaporates using energy, which is costly. Therefore, it is desirable to boil for no longer than necessary, avoid evaporating huge volumes of water, and at least partially recover the energy consumed. Another extremely significant feature of water evaporation is the amount of sparge water that may be used earlier. Consequently, substantial evaporation also increases the yield. Despite the higher yield, it would not be profitable to boil for an extended period since the energy required would be considerably more expensive than the extract's profit (threshold for use of last runnings, Section 1.3.7).

Only water is lost; hence, the amount of extract in the wort must rise. The value is dependent on the process plant that was employed, which corresponds to the various levels of evaporation in various kettles. It rises with the rate of evaporation, and the increase in extract from the raw wort to the finished product might exceed 2%.

The extract concentration of the first wort must be 5–6% greater than the unboiled wort during lautering, as significant dilution takes place during sparging. Evaporation raises the extract content, so again, the final wort has a larger concentration. Similar to the original gravity, the brewery standards for the specific beer type influence the concentration of the pitching wort. The concentration shift that takes place during cooling must also be taken into consideration. The brewing facility determines this modification. Previously, open cooling caused a significant volume of water to evaporate. The extract content rises due to evaporation; it falls due to the addition of sparge water, such as on used hops or other materials. No further evaporation occurs today, and the concentration hardly drops.

Therefore, the extract content must be adjusted at the conclusion of wort boiling to ensure that neither wort cooling changes nor subsequent dilution of the beer by first or final runnings during filtering cause the original wort gravity to drop below the necessary concentration. As a result, efforts are made to maintain the required initial wort gravity content, with a possible variance of 0.1 to 0.3%, depending on brewery requirements. Controlling the extract content is one of the brewhouse manager's most crucial duties. Later, it is quite difficult to fix.

1.3.13 Enzymes Inactivation

The few enzymes that are still present are entirely eliminated during wort boiling. Thus, a subsequent uncontrolled change in the composition of the wort is no longer possible. Malt extract or first wort must be added later to totally decompose the starch to the iodine normal condition or to fermentable sugars when future adjustments are required.

1.3.14 Wort Heating

Boiling causes more tannins to oxidize and more Maillard products and Strecker aldehydes to be produced, increasing the wort's heat exposure and making it darker. As the boiling time increases and the whirlpool rests, the thermal loading, measured in TBI, also increases. Since the TBI also serves as a benchmark for the beer's flavor stability, it is preferable to avoid boiling the beer too vigorously or for an excessively lengthy period of time.

Therefore, modern wort-boiling techniques minimize the temperature exposure. The TBI of the wort (unboiled wort) is around 20–22 and is significantly raised as a result of boiling. The TBI of the cast wort and the TBI of the cold wort after the wort cooler should be below 45 and 60, respectively. During fermentation and maturity, the TBI decreases once again, reaching a value of around 30; however, this number depends on the TBI's peak value, which should be kept as low as possible. As a result, a transient TBI is referred to. However, the TBI of the malt (expressed in the Congress wort) serves as the primary beginning value; therefore it is preferable to maintain a low TBI of the malt.

However, the TBI is not a good direct measure of the beer's flavor stability. For this, the aniline index (Al), which tracks the beer's ageing, especially when kept in warm environments, is measured, or, even better, stability is assessed using an ESR spectrometer.

1.3.15 Wort pH

Since the melanoidins produced while boiling are acidic, and hops also contribute some acid, the wort becomes somewhat more acidic. Unboiled wort has a pH between 5.5 and 5.6 without mash acidification. Cast wort has a pH between 5.4 and 5.5.

At a lower pH, several crucial processes run more smoothly or swiftly. These include a lesser rise in wort color when the pH is lower; better, more flavorful hop bitterness when the pH is lower; and less resistant microorganisms when the pH is lower.

A drawback of adopting a lower pH is that more hops are required since the hop bitter component is used less effectively. Therefore, it is also advisable to biologically acidify the wort to a pH of 5.1–5.2 just before the boiling process is finished.

1.3.16 Reducing Substances (Reductones)

While the wort is boiling, chemicals are created that can interact with the oxygen and have a reducing impact. *Reductones* is the name given to these compounds. These comprise, for instance, melanoidins, the development of which was discussed previously in the section on kilning. The color of the wort grows while boiling and only turns pale once again during fermentation.

1.3.17 Undesirable Aroma Substances

The wort contains a range of more or less volatile aroma substances that have a partly negative effect on the beer's aroma. These undesirable substances include fat-degradation products such as pentanal, hexanal, heptane, and γ-nonalactone, as well as Maillard products and products from the Strecker degradation such as 2- and 3-methyl-butanal, methional, or furfural. The boiling points of these volatile compounds are usually below 100°C, so they evaporate during the wort boiling (Kunze, 2004). Then, in most circumstances, there is a modest increase in the whirlpool, which is frequently greater the quicker the boiling duration. During boiling and heat retention, the amount of substances like furfural, for example, might also rise in some situations. So the TBI and furfural content are related.

It should also be made sure that a 4°C cooling will cut the DMS-P degradation in half. Pre-coolers or strippers can be used to accomplish this.

However, the primary control is focused on thermally separating the DMS precursor and removing the free DMS, which can otherwise impart a vegetable-like flavor and fragrance to beer. Because it is impossible to compensate for insufficient removal of DMS during malt production by boiling in the wort kettle, the maltsters must thoroughly break the precursor and remove the free DMS, as was already described in the kilning. Therefore, it is anticipated that the DMS precursor concentration in the malt would not be higher than 5 mg/kg (5 ppm). The last free DMS must then be removed, if at all possible.

The DMS precursor SMM undergoes more thermal splitting when the wort is cooked for a longer period of time, which also removes more free DMS. After 30 minutes of boiling, the majority of the free DMS has already been relocated. If the boiling period is shortened, a re-formation of free DMS happens at the conclusion of boiling if the thermal splitting of the DMS precursor was inadequate while boiling. The recommendation value for free DMS at the mid-cooling stage is 100 pg/I.

Therefore, it's important to pay attention to getting rid of the later-produced free DMS. This is crucial for stable flavor and a nice beer froth. In any case, it's important to pay attention to evaporation efficiency to avoid flavor flaws in both fresh and aged beer.

Because free DMS can subsequently be generated by thermal splitting above this temperature, the wort must first be cooled to 85°C when employing a pre-cooler between the cast wort and whirlpool.

Plate-type heat exchangers are often used for pre-cooling before the whirlpool, while film evaporators and internal boilers, as well as steam and air strippers, are typically utilized for stripping following the whirlpool. The free DMS that develops during the whirlpool rest is eliminated during stripping.

Even during fermentation, any free DMS that is still present is removed by the fermentation gases. The washing-out effect increases with fermentation temperature but is reduced by counterpressure. The DMS content is decreased by 25% during fermentation.

1.3.18 Whirlpool

The wort is then circulated at high speed to make a whirlpool effect, which leads to coagulation into proteins, enzymes, and residues of hop products.

After 15 to 20 minutes of whirlpool, 10 to 15 minutes of rest is given. Coagulated matter will settle out of the liquid as a sludge that is called trub.

Trub is partially removed from the bottom of the whirlpool kettle, which ensures the bitter wort is clear when transferred to the next step.

1.3.19 Chilling

After the whirlpool rest, the wort is cooled to around 10–20°C (depends on styles) through a heat exchanger on its way to the fermenter. This process takes about an hour.

Temperature of wort chilling varies depending on beer styles: for example, for lagers, it's 10°C; for ales, it's 18–22°C.

By heat exchanging, we recover the energy used to boil the wort: i.e., cold water becomes hot water and is returned to the hot liquor tank and is then used to brew more beer or for cleaning.

1.3.20 Fermentation

After wort chilling, the yeast is pitched. The wort will be fermented by yeast, which coverts it into beer.

Primary fermentation takes three to four days. Fermentation temperatures vary, depending on beer styles: for a lager, its below 12°C; ales are fermented above 20°C.

1.3.21 Maturation

At the end of fermentation, the finished beer is chilled to 8°C and then to 4°C and is kept in the tank for maturation at 1°C for 15 to 25 days.

Conical fermenters are used for fermentation, and yeast is harvested from the cone at the bottom of the fermenter and can be pitched to new batch of beer.

1.3.22 Packaging

The beer is then filtered into a bright beer tank (BBT) when it has to be packaged, either in kegs or in bottles. Diatomaceous earth is used as the filtration medium. It filters out yeast and other particulates and clarifies the beer.

The carbon dioxide (CO_2) is adjusted in the BBT, and the beer is then ready to be packaged. Beer is kept freezing cold. Beer is either packaged into kegs (20 ltr) or bottled in 330 mL glass bottles.

If the beer is being bottled, it is counter-pressure filled (double pre-evacuation) to lessen oxidation and capped on froth to make sure there are no undesirable bacteria and that it will stay stable in the bottle.

1.3.23 Serving

Kegs are delivered to bars and pubs and also used for festivals and promotions. Bottles are delivered to off-licenses, restaurants, pubs, sporting clubs, etc.

1.4 IMPLICATIONS AND BENEFITS OF BEER

As a "greenhouse gas," CO_2 has the potential to harm the environment as a significant fermentation product. Because the fermentation process only operates at a low head pressure, some of the CO_2 generated does not remain dissolved in the beer. (High CO_2 concentrations in the fermenting beer can have adverse effects on yeast performance and the production of flavor components, such as esters.) Instead of letting the extra CO_2 leak into the environment, it is collected from the top of the fermenting containers. The CO_2 is "scrubbed" to eliminate contaminants, and the excess may be sold to gas providers for a profit or, in certain circumstances, fed back into the completed product to increase the amount of carbonation (Campbell, 2017). The continuous fermenter prevents losses (lower wastage) brought on by stop-start operations from occurring. To remove any remaining beer, surplus yeast from the fermenter is collected and rinsed counter currently with de-aerated water. The fermented beer is then diluted with the water that contains beer extracts, and the yeast is marketed as a food ingredient. Extra CO_2 is collected, cleaned, and perhaps utilized again. In further steps of the process, CO_2 can be utilized from fermenter for a constant supply of CO_2. Since the fermentation process requires only five containers, less money is spent on energy, labor, and testing (Campbell, 2017).

1.5 HEALTH BENEFITS OF BEER

If beer is consumed in moderation, it provides several health advantages. The following are a few of these intriguing health advantages (Ore et al., 2018).

Anti-cancer attributes: The flavonoid xanthohumol found in beer-making hops is important in the chemoprevention of cancer, particularly prostate cancer.

Decreased risk of heart disease: Vitamin B6, which is found in beer, guards against heart problems by inhibiting the buildup of a substance called homocysteine. The line-Beer drinking reduces the risk of fractures and osteoporosis through increasing bone density, must be placed in Osteoporosis and kidney stones section.

Diabetes: A low prevalence of type 2 diabetes is associated with moderate beer intake.

Avoidance of anemia: Beer is a rich source of folic acid and vitamin B12, which prevent anaemia. Additionally, vitamin B12 is necessary for supporting healthy development, sharp memory, and attention.

Hypertension: Regular beer consumers have lower blood pressure than those who regularly consume wine or other alcoholic beverages, according to biomedicine.

Anti-ageing characteristics: Vitamin E, a significant antioxidant in the body, is strengthened and has a greater effect when consumed with beer. It plays a crucial role in maintaining healthy skin and slowing down the ageing process.

Gallstones: Regular moderate beer drinking lowers bile concentration and affects cholesterol levels, which lowers the likelihood of gallstone development.

Prevention of coronary disease and dementia: Additionally, drinking beer increases "good" cholesterol levels by 10–20%, lowering the risk of dementia and cardiovascular illnesses.

Digestive system: Beer has a variety of digestive effects, including the activation of pancreatic enzymes, gastrin, gastric acid, and cholecystokinin.

Osteoporosis and kidney stones: Beer's potassium, sodium, and magnesium content are crucial in lowering the incidence of kidney stones. Beer also contains silicon, which is easily absorbed by the body and further explains why beer has an anti-osteoporosis effect.

Stress relief: Like other alcoholic beverages, beer helps with sleep and reduces stress.

Beer also has a diuretic effect and greatly increases urination. This makes it easier for the body to remove more waste products and pollutants.

1.6 REFERENCES

Aroh, K. (2019). Beer production. *SSRN Electronic Journal*. https://doi.org/10.2139/ssrn.34589833458983

Bokulich, N. A., & Bamforth, C. W. (2013). The microbiology of malting and brewing. *Microbiology and Molecular Biology Reviews*, *77*(2), 157–172.

Campbell, S. L. (2017). *The continuous brewing of beer*. DB Breweries Ltd.

De Keukeleire, D. (2000). Fundamentals of beer and hop chemistry. *Quimica Nova*, *23*, 108–112.

Eaton, B. (2017). An overview of brewing. In *Handbook of brewing* (pp. 53–66). CRC Press.

Hough, J. S., Briggs, D. E., Stevens, R., & Young, T. W. (1982). Chemical and physical properties of beer. In *Malting and brewing science* (pp. 776–838). Springer.

Kunze, W. (2004). *Brewing malting* (pp. 18–152). VLB.

Ore, G., Mironov, M., & Shootov, A. (2018). Design and production of maize beer. *International Journal of Food Processing Technology*, *6*, 78–87.

Sánchez, H. C. (2017). The mathematics of brewing. Available @http://chalkdustmagazine.com/blog/the-mathematics-of-brewing/

Stewart, G. G. (2016). Saccharomyces species in the production of beer. *Beverages*, *2*(4), 34.

Wong, G. (2003). Role of yeast in production of alcoholic beverage. *Botany*, *135*(1), 30–45.

2 Historical Concept of Brewing

One of the first known drinks in human history is beer. The earliest known written record is a clay tablet from the Sumerian civilization that depicts the making of alcohol and is thought to be roughly 6,000 years old. In ancient civilizations, beer was extensively consumed and had a big impact on society.

Beer was literally "the nectar of the gods," emerging onto the global scene in the Fertile Crescent as a sacred beverage, according to the earliest inscriptions we have about it. The world's earliest civilizations made beer and spoke extensively about it, providing an intriguing historical trail for us to interpret and comprehend.

One of the oldest beverages ever made by humans is beer. It is thought that the first beer was produced in prehistoric Mesopotamia (present-day Iraq, Iran, Syria, and portions of Turkey) between 10,000 and 5000 BCE. Additionally, because microorganisms were eliminated during the boiling process, it was commonly believed to be safer and healthier to consume than water.

Additionally, it had nutrients that earlier beverages lacked. However, as the Mesopotamians were not big on recording everything, there is no written evidence of the exact date when beer was first produced. The ancient Egyptians were the first to record their beer formula. Their beer recipe is really the oldest known recipe for any meal or drink in the entire world (Hornsey, 2003).

The ancient Sumerians also used to worship beer. Ninkasi was known as the goddess of beer, and one of the poems was written about her around 1800 BCE includes a recipe for beer. There is a 3,900-year-old Sumerian poem called "The Hymn to Ninkasi" that describes how beer was made from bread and barley. "The Hymn to Ninkasi," written on a stone tablet is regarded as one of the oldest beer recipes. Straws were used by the Sumerians and Egyptians as sediment filters. The straw was only utilized during the sipping process—not while the beer was being brewed. Depending on the social standing of the drinker, straws of the period were either made of reeds or of gold (Cabras & Higgins, 2016).

The Sumerian recipe for beer eventually made its way to ancient Egypt, where it flourished. Many individuals still hold the belief that ancient Egyptian beer would have been similar to porridge and consumed with straws, exactly like Sumerian and Natufian beer. However, a team from the British Museum sought to reproduce the beer using authentic formulas, and were shocked to discover that it tasted just like today's beer.

To hasten the fermenting process, the ancient Egyptians would have used dates, spices, seeds, flower petals, and other ingredients. We should emphasize that the British Museum team's educated guesses are all that they had to go on, but the procedure does seem to be effective. The Egyptian beverage was considerably different from the Sumerian beer, which was consumed using a straw from a big bowl (to avoid

DOI: 10.1201/b22906-2

ingesting the mash). The ladies of the household would brew beer at home, but the Egyptians were the first to establish state-owned breweries. The beer produced at these breweries was utilized for celebrations (where it was frequently distributed gratis) and was also distributed to employees (such as to the men that built the pyramids) (Hornsey, 2003).

However, the Egyptians produced a variety of beers. They drank their typical beer, which tasted like brown ales. Then, they had a lager-like lighter beer (served on special occasions), higher-alcohol brews (served at funerals), and beer with honey added to it. Only the pharaoh and his household/guests were permitted to use this last one.

The pharaohs set the brewing schedules and oversaw the distribution methods, with the Egyptians primarily using beer in religious rites. Beer was also utilized by the Egyptians for medicinal purposes and as part of the burial supplies needed for the transition to the next life.

Egyptian beer has been discussed in many other nations; the ancient Greeks and Romans also wrote about it. Although it was produced in both ancient Greece and Rome, beer was never as well liked as wine. However, the Romans helped disseminate beer throughout their empire and developed a more industrialized brewing method. It is believed that during the Roman rule, beer was imported to Britain.

When the Babylonians conquered Sumer, they were quick to adopt the superior beer-making skills of the Sumerians. The Babylonian king, Hammurabi, even categorized beer into 20 different varieties. For instance, there are a few passages pertaining to beer and its manufacture in Hammurabi's legislation. Beer was also immensely popular in Egypt, and archaeologists discovered the oldest brewery in the world that has been maintained to the present day at Nekhen (also known as Hierakonpolis). In Tell el-Farkha, archaeologists from Poland, under the direction of Professor Krzysztof Ciaowicz from Jagiellonian University, uncovered a sizable complex made up of six breweries that was roughly a century younger than the one unearthed in Nekhen. There are still theories that these breweries were constructed on the foundations of earlier ones (Jackowski & Trusek, 2018).

As the Greek empire expanded, they initially continued to prefer their wine over beer. Eventually, even they included beer in their diet. The Greek writer Sophocles said that the best diet consisted of bread, meats, vegetables, and beer.

During the Middle Ages and the Dark Ages, beer would become extremely popular in Europe. While the days of Egypt's beer production had ended, the spread of Islam, which outlawed alcohol, put an end to it. Regrettably, for centuries, beer was not brewed in Egypt, Iraq, Iran, Israel, Jordan, etc. Some Middle Eastern nations continue to lack a beer industry.

Europe was left to its own devices and divided into smaller nations after the Roman Empire crumbled. The term "Dark Ages" is also used to describe this time period, but it has less and less support. It is unquestionably true that many of the inventions the Romans brought with them were forgotten and needed to be learned again centuries later.

During the Middle Ages, the majority of beer was made at home, while several monasteries produced wine or beer for sale. The beer and ale would have been comparable to Egyptian brews: just grains, water, and wild yeast—no hops—with of fruits, nuts, and spices to add flavor (or increase alcohol by volume) (Hornsey, 2003).

The Roman Empire was no longer able to defend the population after its demise. Law and order were destroyed, which resulted in the feudal system that offered some measure of safety and defense. In the Middle Ages, the Church had a significant role in defending alcohol.

The primary hubs for brewing and wine-making expertise after the fall of the Roman Empire were monasteries (monks). Domestic brewing of rural brews continued. However, monks virtually took over the craft of brewing. And they protected their wisdom with great care. Up until the 12th century, almost all high-quality beer was produced by monks. The monks were therefore a major source of alcohol during the Middle Ages. In the Middle Ages, monks continued to cultivate vineyards. They possessed the means, safety, and stability needed to gradually raise the caliber of their vines. The monks also had the training and leisure to improve their knowledge of viticulture. Consequently, monks owned and managed the best vineyards during the Middle Ages. Wine was obviously required to celebrate mass. To maintain themselves, the monks generated a lot as well (Hornsey, 2003).

Mead, rustic brews, and wild fruit wines rose in popularity in the early Middle Ages. The Celts, Anglo-Saxons, Germans, and Scandinavians were most affected by this. However, in the nations of the Romance Age, wine remained the favored libation. Tithes, sales, and taxes might all be paid in beer.

In feudal England, very few commoners had ever tried claret (red Bordeaux wine). Ale was a staple meal for them rather than a beverage. Surprisingly, everyone had ale for breakfast—adults and children—in addition to their midday meal and, finally, just before they turned in for the night (Donnachie, 1979).

Barley was a typical grain in many Mediterranean societies. It flourished in that setting and was used as the main ingredient in a variety of breads and cakes. People quickly learned that wetting barley, letting it germinate (form sprouts), and then drying it would produce a sweeter, less perishable grain.

Meanwhile, in China, beer was brewed using millet, barley, and tubers. According to historians, central China was first introduced to barley for the purpose of brewing beer. Further evidence from archaeology indicates that the Chinese produced beer around 7000 BCE using a method quite similar to that of the ancient Mesopotamians and Egyptians. However, the Elba tablets reveal that beer was made in Syria as early as 2500 BCE.

A few regions of Northern Europe started growing hops about the 9th century. Hops would certainly have been added to beers as early as then in places like Bavaria. Hops imparted a bitter flavor to the beer while also extending its shelf life. Beer would seldom have been allowed to mature for a long time until hops started to be used regularly. Compared to the beer today, the majority of it would be quite "young."

A little Irish tavern was opening its doors at the same time as Bavarians were experimenting with hops. In 900 AD, Sean's Bar in Athlone first opened. Hops may have been introduced to beer by Bavarians as early as the middle of the 7th century. But it's not known when or where hop-infused brewing first began. Hopped beer was a brand new alcoholic beverage. The sole ingredients used in its exact fermentation were water, barley, and hops. It's important to note that adding hops produced good taste and preservation. In the Middle Ages, alcohol saw significant development due to the utilization of hops. Poppy seeds, mushrooms, aromatics, honey, sugar, bay leaves, butter, and bread crumbs were among the components used in early recipes (Hornsey, 2003).

The St. Gall monastery established Switzerland's first significant brewery. Each monk at the time received five quarts of beer every day. Alcohol had a major role in Viking society. Their gods were heavy drinkers. In their ideal world, heroes who had died could continue to fight for all eternity on a battlefield. Its celebration area was called Valhalla. Every night, the departed went there to eat roast pig and mead. The best part was that stunning blonde Valkyries served it. The Vikings drank beer, mead, ale, and wine. They preferred ale, but they also enjoyed mead. A powerful (9% alcohol) black, sweet, malty beverage was produced in an attempt to replicate a Viking brew. In a time when sugar was scarce, it would have felt much sweeter. Before serving, the Vikings strained the brew. We are aware of this because ale strainers have been found in tombs by archaeologists. Records indicate that hop farming thrived in Bohemia (Meussdoerffer, 2009).

After the ninth century, hops began to be used extensively. For over 500 years, the term "beer" was absent from the English language. Perhaps this was due to beer being a stronger, more costly, upper-class beverage than ale (Donnachie, 1979).

Weihenstefan Abbey began manufacturing beer in the 11th century; the brewery is still in use today, making it one of the world's oldest corporations. The beer created in the 11th century could have had hops, but it might also have been brewed similarly to the majority of beers at the time (without hops and with flavorings like fruit, seeds, and spices).

In England, alewives made at least two different strengths of beer, whereas monks brewed three. They used "single," "double," or "triple" to indicate how strong the liquor was. In England, Anselm ruled that priests shouldn't partake in excessive drinking or attend drinking events. The first national tax on beer in England was enacted in 1188 to fund the Crusades. Hops started to appear often in various beers during the 13th century, notably in northern Europe, for flavoring and preservation. Ale was frequently a filling, soup-like beverage. Ale was brewed for local consumption only. It immediately became sour because of the absence of hops (Donnachie, 1979).

Thousands of brewsters met the enormous demand for ale in England. Women made up the bulk of them; it was one of the few trades available to women in mediaeval times. According to King Henry III in 1267, "Ale was so essential to commoners for basic survival that why its price and quality were governed by legislation." In England, there were three different types of public locations where individuals could purchase alcohol: (1) alehouses, (2) taverns that served wine in addition to beer, and (3) inns that also accommodated pilgrims (Donnachie, 1979).

The most well-liked type of celebration in England around the turn of the century was ale. Beer and ale were popular forms of rent payment among lords. German towns enjoyed the prerogative of making and selling beer in their immediate communities as they arose in the 11th century. Craft brewing became a thriving industry in many communities, and municipal pride was high. Due to the usage of hops by its brewers, Hamburg experienced a thriving alcohol trade during the 1200s. With the introduction of new apple types, hard or fermented cider consumption grew in popularity in England in the middle of the 1200s (Donnachie, 1979).

England was a major wine producer before 1300. The majority of Northern Europe and all of Southern Europe would have consumed more of it. Wineries collapsed as a result of the chilly weather; therefore, Northern European nations switched to lager.

Obviously, these events have been greatly simplified. Germany continued to manufacture wine at that time, England was already importing French wine, and France continued to make wine throughout the Middle Ages. Climate change undoubtedly had an impact on beer production, but it was just one of several.

During the period from 1315 to 1898, the world's climate underwent a significant transformation; the Little Ice Age was in effect. From around 1560 to 1660, it was very bad. All forms of agriculture, including viniculture, were severely disrupted by the Little Ice Age. As a result, wine was hard to come by.

The start of the Little Ice Age was followed by the Black Death and other epidemics, which decreased the population by as much as 82% in some communities. There were folks that significantly increased their alcohol intake, believing it might shield them from the unknown illness. Others believed they could be protected by using moderation in everything, including drinking. Overall, it would seem that alcohol consumption was high. For instance, the average annual beer intake in Bavaria was probably around 300 liters. That is equivalent to around 150 liters now. Each person in Florence consumed around 10 barrels of wine annually. Additionally, there was an upsurge in the use of distilled spirits for medical purposes. One or two gallons of ale consumed daily by adult males was not unusual in Britain in the 1300s, according to one historian. As the Middle Ages came to a conclusion, beer became increasingly popular in Scotland, England, and France. By the end of the Middle Ages, people began to use spirits as a beverage. Over 60% of families in one English community made a living from the production or sale of ale. One alcohol seller was reportedly present for every 12 people in 1309 London. A proclamation was issued limiting the use of wheat in brewing because of a grain shortage in England. In mediaeval Scotland, adulterating alcoholic liquids was a capital offense.

Wine and beer were to be sold for a fair price under an English law. But there was no explanation of how to figure out what a fair price might be. A French statute mandated that bars provide wine upon request. Florence forbade innkeepers from selling wine or other alcoholic beverages to the underprivileged in 1357. A royal permit was necessary to export English beer and ale in 1366. In 1381, when the price of maize rose in England, so did the cost of ale. This raised worries that the underprivileged wouldn't be able to purchase it. As a result, the London mayor enacted price caps on beer. Duke Philip the Bold set regulations controlling Burgundy wine production in 1395 to raise the quality. He gave the order to demolish all Gamay-planted vines. In his words, the "disloyal plant produces a wine in tremendous quantity but horrendous in harshness."

Between 1396 and 1878, when the Turks imposed Muslim control, wine making in Bulgaria came to an end. The Middle Ages had their share of alcoholic beverages.

2.1 THE RENAISSANCE (1400–1618)

The era up to the Industrial Revolution witnessed the most significant developments in beer manufacturing and culture. It is the matter to understand that how much beer evolved as a beverage between 1400 and 1618, the period that most historians think of as the Renaissance.

The majority of beer was brewed at home in 1400, fermented for a short period of time, and manufactured without the use of hops. Things started to shift about the year 1480. In 1487, the Munich beer rules were introduced, and two years later, Germany's first brewing guild was established. In London, the first brewer's guild was established in 1493.

In the 1490s, Columbus claimed to have seen Indians brewing beer from corn and black birch sap. The early colonists' claims that they brought the first beers to the Americas were refuted by this. However, the first permanent structure constructed at Plymouth Rock by the pilgrims was a brewery.

By today's standards, the 16th century had an extremely high level of beer consumption. In addition, there was more regulation during that time. Such laws were intended to guarantee the quality of the beer, the livelihood of the workforce, fire safety, and high tax collections, not to cut down on consumption.

In Coventry, a person would typically drink 17 pints of beer or ale every week. That is equivalent to around three pints in modern-day England. The average daily intake across the nation was one pint per person. Each day, soldiers were given two-thirds of a gallon of beer. Peasants in Poland drank up to three liters of beer per day. The amount of beer consumed in Sweden may have been 40 times what it is now. For adult laborers and sailors in Denmark, a gallon of beer was typically consumed each day.

2.2 *REINHEITSGEBOT* (GERMAN PURITY LAW)

In Bavaria, the *Reinheitsgebot*, or legislation on the purity of beer, was established. The *Reinheitsgebot* was initially put into effect in 1516. The Bavarian brewing guilds had pushed it. Several variants of this regulation were already in place in many German towns and cities. These statutes, however, are the most well known and are still in force today. The only ingredients allowed for the production of beer are barley, water, and hops. Yeast was not addressed, although this was mainly due to the fact that at the time, it was not well known.

Although there were other reasons, the German Purity Law was primarily intended to raise beer quality. To avoid rivalry with bakers and maintain cheap pricing, barley was promoted above other grains. Another objective was to lessen competition from Northern and Eastern German brewers, who frequently added other ingredients to their beer.

The laws are frequently believed to be the same today, however this couldn't be farther from the reality. Just a few years later, wheat was added to the list of permitted substances. Yeast was also included. Over time, other ingredients were added, and more are still being introduced so that Germany doesn't fall behind in the craft beer movement.

The laws were very beneficial to Germany at the time and have advanced brewing internationally. But compared to nations like Belgium, there is a sense that Germany has lagged behind a little because of the legislation.

2.3 ENGLISH HOPS

English brewers sought to avoid using hops until around 1520, when they started to grow their own. But finally, brewers gave up, and English beer underwent a permanent transformation. Un-hopped beers were becoming increasingly difficult to get in Europe at this time. Scottish "heather" beers as well as comparable beverages in England, Belgium, Holland, Germany, and Ireland started to disappear.

Hops were simply too delicious to pass up. They assisted in keeping the beer fresher for a longer period of time, allowing it to travel farther and acquire superior flavor over time. Additionally, hops offered a fantastic flavor all on their own, making it no longer necessary to utilize pricey spices.

In order to boost the scale of commercial breweries, Denmark set minimal standards. This was done to make tax collection easier. Additionally, it lessened the risk of fires. Making one's own barrels was forbidden for breweries in England. This was done to save the coopers' way of life. Brandenberg outlawed illegal brewing in 1536 to save the local economy, which depended on beer sales. Of course, it also helped raise tax income. Brandenberg forbade the production and serving of alcohol on Sundays and other holidays in 1540. German merchants began offering beer in glass bottles around 1561. As Puritanism developed, there were more assaults on inebriation and alehouses. A gallon of beer was provided as part of each seaman's daily ration in the English navy.

2.4 COLONIAL BEER

The first beers were also made in nations that had been colonized by European powers during the Renaissance. When Sir Walter Raleigh founded a colony in Virginia in 1587, beer was made for the first time in America. The *Mayflower*'s journey may have been impacted by the availability of beer.

When Cortes and his troops conquered Mexico in 1520, beer was first brought to the country. In Mexico, the first brewery was established in 1544.

Strong ale was the breakfast beverage of English Queen Elizabeth I. Ivan the Terrible, the tsar of Russia, switched state-run pubs from selling beer to vodka. At Sir Walter Raleigh's colony in Virginia, the first beer made in the New World was produced. However, it wasn't warmly received by the colonists. They wanted English beer. Men and women who were held accountable for issues with brewing were known as "brew witches" or "beer witches." In the 16th century, such executions were an unpleasant aspect of beer.

In 1600, the Dutch briefly introduced beer to Japan by opening a beer hall in Nagasaki. But this brief dalliance with beer was abruptly ended, and the Dutch were expelled.

2.5 17TH CENTURY

In the 17th century, little changed in the beer world. Due to advancements in transportation, beer could now be delivered all the way to the New World. Additionally, there were both technical and legal breakthroughs. But there were several modifications in the 18th century. After the Industrial Revolution changed the way malt was dried, England also created pale ale and later India pale ale.

Brewing beer was one of colonial North America's first businesses. Hops were first grown in the Massachusetts Colony. In the colony of Maryland, laws supported brewing. The Kalevala saga of Finland was recorded through oral tradition. It talks about producing beer utilizing hops. Ale could be kept fresher for a longer period of time in glass bottles with cork closures, as observed by Dr. Alexander Nowell, the dean of St. Paul's Cathedral in 1602 (Mittelman, 2008).

The first supply of English beer came to the colony of Virginia in 1607. A brewer was sought by the colonists of Virginia in London in 1609. On the southernmost point of New Amsterdam, the first brewery was recorded in the New World.

A malt tax was introduced in England. In North America, the first non-native was born. The location was a brewery. The youngster, Jean Vigne, went on to establish himself as the first brewer to be born in the New World. The *Mayflower* brought the Pilgrims to Plymouth in the Massachusetts Colony in 1620. On board, there was a severe shortage of beer, so the crew members had the passengers get off the ship to guarantee they would have enough beer for their journey back to England (Donnachie, 1979).

Ireland started giving licenses to alcoholic beverage merchants in 1634. The first brewery was established in the Massachusetts Colony. Boston issued a bar license in 1637. Levies on beer were first implemented by the English Parliament in 1643. Its goal was to raise money to fight the Crown.

The Netherlands and France each had a portion of the Caribbean island of St. Martin. The northern portion was given to France as "Saint Martin." The Netherlands received the southern portion as "Saint Maarten." A Frenchman and a Dutchman are said to have stood side by side in the island's middle, according to folklore. Then, they walked away with their shares. The Dutchman frequently paused to sip beer. As a result, a smaller portion of the island was given to the Netherlands.

A law authorizing the export of "Beer, Ale, and Mum" was enacted by King Charles II of England in 1671. Dublin had 91 public houses, 1,180 alehouses, and around 4,000 households. Harvard College had its own brewhouse in 1674 to guarantee that there would be enough high-quality beer for the pupils. In the 1680s, England's preferred beverage was beer. Throughout the decade, consumption increased to 104 gallons per person overall. Pennsylvania was established in 1680 by William Penn, who also established a commercial brewery there (Donnachie, 1979).

The pint (568 milliliters) became a standard unit of measurement in Britain around 1698. This amount of pour eventually became the norm for beer and cider. Pubs were only permitted to offer beer in a pint, a third, or half of that measurement (Donnachie, 1979).

2.6 18TH-CENTURY BREWERIES

In the 18th century, beer's history was essentially one of invention. With the creation and advancement of the steam engine, beer production became industrialized. Improvements to brewing techniques also received more attention over the century.

Every few days, women in the northern colonies of what is now the United States made beer. Their drink only lasted a short time. John Clarke, a Londoner, created the hydrometer in 1730, which calculated the amount of alcohol in beer. In the 1740s, there were 100 breweries in the Netherlands that employed 1,200 people.

The earliest documented brewster in North America was Mary Lisle in 1734. She took over running her late father's Philadelphia brewery. Numerous renowned breweries were established throughout the 18th century all across the world. Guinness is a beverage that originated in the Irish village of Leixlip. Arthur Guinness started brewing a dark-brown stout in 1755. George Washington penned his own recipe for "To Make Small Beer" in 1757. It was an early attempt to develop guidelines and norms for the craft of brewing. The Warsteiner Brewery was established in 1753, while the Rothaus Brewery in Germany first opened its doors in 1791. The Whitbread and Courage Breweries were established in London in the 18th century as well (Mittelman, 2008).

Frederick II, the Prussian monarch, increased the price of coffee in 1763. He wanted to expand his brewing business since it brought in a lot of money. Industrialization of beer became a reality with the introduction of the steam engine in 1765. At Fort Pitt (Pittsburgh, PA), the British Army constructed the first brewery west of the Allegheny Mountains.

In 1767, a British businessman made a deal with the East India Company to supply beer to the British merchants and civil service in the India colonies. To help the beer last on its lengthy journey, he doubled the hop level. In England, porter, a blend of dark and light malts, was created in 1772. One quart of hard cider or spruce beer was rationed to each soldier each day during the Revolutionary War in 1775 by Congress. Charles Hall started a brewery in Dorset, England, in 1777. The Hall & Woodhouse Brewery was established in 1847 when the Woodhouses mated into the family (Donnachie, 1979).

In 1783, John H. Molson bought a stake in a brewery housed in a log cabin along the St. Lawrence River in what is now Canada. The empire of Molson Beer started with this. Both Thomas Jefferson and George Washington had their own personal breweries. Samuel Adams ran a for-profit brewery. Joseph Bramah, a British inventor, filed a patent for a beer-pump handle in 1785. In Canada, the Molson Brewery (now Molson-Coors) was established in 1786. James Madison suggested a low tariff on domestic beer in 1789 to promote its manufacture.

A statute encouraging the production and consumption of beer and ale was approved in Massachusetts. George Washington said he would only drink porter produced in the United States. In 1789, New Hampshire opted not to impose a tax on brewing property

2.7 19TH-CENTURY BREWERIES

One of the most fascinating eras in the history of beer making is the 19th century. This century saw the true globalization of beer as several nations established their own breweries. In 1805, hops were first grown in Australia. Oktoberfest began around 1810 in Munich, Germany.

In the United States, 185,000 barrels of beer were produced by 132 breweries. Seven million people made up the nation's population. The *American Brewer and Maltster* first appeared in print in 1815. The drum roaster's introduction in 1817 made it possible to produce malts that were extremely black and roasted. Porters and stouts benefited from this in terms of flavor.

A Philadelphia brewery constructed a steam engine in 1818. This was the first engine utilized in the brewing of beer in North America. In Pottsville, Pennsylvania, The Yuengling Brewery started making beer in 1829. The Yuengling family still owns the oldest brewery in the United States. The 1830 Beer Act was adopted in England, and a ratepayer was able to purchase a license to brew and sell beer. Belgium resisted the Netherlands. The high beer tariffs were one of the causes of the uprising. The largest brewery in Ireland in 1833 was called Guinness.

Belgian Trappist monks of St. Sixtus started making Westvleteren Beer in 1839 to pay for a new monastery. By 1844, a Bavarian brewmaster in Pilsen, Bohemia (Czech Republic), had invented pilsner. In Milwaukee, a brewery that would later become Pabst Brewing was founded. Carlsberg started brewing beer in Denmark in 1847. Milwaukee saw the establishment of a brewery in 1849, which later became the Schlitz Brewery.

In the United States, 750,000 barrels of beer (31 gallons per barrel) were produced by 431 breweries in 1850. Over a million barrels of beer were produced in the United States by a total of 1,269 breweries in 1860; 85% of the total was generated in New York and Pennsylvania. The first refrigeration device used for commerce was granted a US patent. Later, this turned out to be crucial for the manufacture and distribution of beer (Mittelman, 2008).

For the duration of the American Civil War (1861–1865), beer was subject to a $1-per-barrel levy. Gerard Adriaan Heineken established a brewery in Amsterdam, the Netherlands, in 1864. After the American Civil War, beer became the favorite libation of working men instead of whiskey. Six million barrels of beer were produced in the United States in 1867 (Mittelman, 2008).

The first issue of the monthly publication The *American Brewer* was published in 1868, the same year John Siebel founded a brewing school that would eventually become the Siebel Institute of Technology.

Adolphus Busch invented the usage of double-walled railcars in the 1870s. They received their supplies from a system of icehouses. Budweiser was able to do this and eventually become the first national beer brand. Anheuser registered the "A and eagle" trademark in 1872. New York City saw the first strike by brewery employees.

Germany's Beck's Brewery was established in Bremen in 1873. Nine million barrels of beer were produced in the United States by a record 4,131 breweries. In Singen, Thuringia, Germany, an innkeeper constructed the Schmitt Brewery for his eatery. *Studies on Fermentation*, written by Louis Pasteur, described the function of yeast in brewing in 1876. To stabilize beer, he created the pasteurization procedure 22 years before milk was pasteurized.

The Guinness Brewery expanded to become the biggest on the globe in 1880. A German inventor created a beer filter in 1880. Frederick Salem wrote a book titled *Beer, Its History and Its Economic Value as a National Beverage*. He made the case that drinking beer was a successful method of maintaining one's temper. His catchphrase was "Beer versus whisky." In the United States, there were 2,830 breweries, and the American Brewers Academy was established in 1880.

In the United States, the National Brewers' and Distillers' Association was established in 1882. Denmark is where the first single-cell yeast culture was discovered in 1883. The best strains of yeast might then be chosen by brewers. Removing undesired yeast strains also improved brand consistency. In Juneau, Alaska, the first brewery opened in 1886.

Brewery employees went on strike in New York, Chicago, and Milwaukee in 1887. The Master Brewer's Association was established. A brewer volunteered to pump his beer into a fountain in Portland, Oregon, for its dedication in 1888. The city turned down the proposal. Pabst was the first American brewer to sell more than a million barrels in a calendar year in the 1890s. Philippine brewer San Miguel first produced beer in 1890 (Mittelman, 2008).

The wood pulp coaster was created in Dresden, Germany, in 1892, while the crown top was created in Baltimore. South African Breweries (SAB) was established in 1895. During the Spanish-American War in 1898, the United States increased the beer barrel tax to $2.00, and beer sales decreased as a result. The Royal Brewery was Hawaii's first brewery in 1898.

2.8 1900 TO THE PRESENT

Numerous modifications were made to beer's history over the 20th century. Beer experienced some strange times at the start of the 20th century. Numerous developments occurred in terms of laws, technology, science, corporate structure, and other factors. They had an impact on brewing methods, the size of the brewery, drink preferences, and drinking habits. Homebrewing, microbreweries, and brew pubs are all currently expanding, reflecting these developments.

While several nations built their first breweries, others started to oppose it. Although the temperance movement had existed since the late 18th century, it only really took off in the 20th century. The United States and several Scandinavian nations both outlawed alcohol, which caused all American breweries to close, completely altering the beer scene (Mittelman, 2008).

The two World Wars also had a significant impact on beer. Before World War II, Nazi meetings took place often in German beer halls, and the conflict had an adverse effect on a number of breweries. After World War II, the Soviet Union closed down breweries at will, thereby destroying East Germany's beer culture (Meussdoerffer, 2009).

The emergence of the major six breweries that effectively controlled the entire beer market in England had an impact on the beer scene in Britain. The communist regime nationalized every brewery in Poland (Szymczak, 2019).

In 1901, the United States decreased the levy on a barrel of beer from $2.00 to $1.60. Busch surpassed Pabst to become the most popular beer in the country. The United States lowered the beer barrel tax to $1.00 in 1902. Tsingtao Brewery was established in China in 1903 by German brewers, and the first completely mechanized bottle-making equipment was created.

Teddy Roosevelt took more than 500 liters of alcohol on an African safari in 1909. The Webb-Kenyon Act was approved by Congress in 1913. It forbade the delivery of alcoholic drinks into the United States. The prohibition of alcohol on American naval sites and ships was issued by the Secretary of the Navy in 1914.

In order to conserve grain for the war effort, President Woodrow Wilson ordered the closure of all U.S. breweries in 1918. The 18th Amendment to the United States Constitution was passed by Congress in January 1919. It stipulated that the National Prohibition Act would start one year after the ratification date. This was a significant occasion in 20th-century beer history.

For the purpose of establishing National Prohibition, Congress approved the Volstead Act in 1921. During Prohibition (1920–1933), brewers developed "near beers" with an alcohol content of less than 0.5%. The brands included Pablo by Pabst, Famo by Schlitz, Miller's Vivo, Stroh's Lux-O, and Busch's Anheuser-Bevo. The Willis Campbell Act was approved by President Warren G. Harding. The measure was sometimes referred to as the *anti-beer law*. It made it illegal for doctors to recommend beer as a medication. Wine and alcoholic beverages were allowed, nevertheless (Meussdoerffer, 2009).

National Prohibition faced increasing opposition in 1926. According to a national poll on prohibition, respondents were nine to one in support of either its modification or its repeal. According to the Association Against the Prohibition Amendment, in 1928, enough hops were sold during the course of the year to produce 20 million barrels of illicit beer. One argument they used to abolish Prohibition was the loss of revenue from these sales.

Breweries in the United States sold 86 million gallons of near beer in total in 1932. Congress amended the Volstead Act with the Cullen-Harrison Act because it was anticipated that it would take years to eliminate national prohibition. That authorized the sale of 3.2% alcohol beer and wine. The goal was to swiftly boost both employment and tax income. The law went into force on April 7, 1933. Thirty-one breweries had resumed operations by June (Mittelman, 2008). Another significant development in the history of beer in the 20th century was this: It is now National Beer Day on April 7.

The introduction of the beer can in 1933 in the United States led to an increase in home beer consumption. British beer drinkers preferred mild ale and bitter and also from the increasing numbers of home refrigerators led to an increase in beer consumption at home. In 1934, 756 breweries were operating again as a result of the repeal of Prohibition.

The majority of drinking in the Netherlands occurred in bars up until 1940. After that, drinking at home was commonplace. Pre-prohibition levels of beer output were attained. However, there were just half as many breweries in business as there were in 1910. In the United States, the barrel tax was increased from $5.00 to $6.00. In 1943, the United States required breweries to set aside 15% of their output for military use. The US barrel tax was increased from $6.00 to $8.00. Max Heinrich, a German brewer, created Zambia's Chibuku beer in the 1950s.

The US barrel tax was increased to $9.00 in 1951. Morton W. Coutts, a New Zealander, developed the continuous fermentation method in 1953. His method prevents beer from ever being exposed to the environment before the bottle is opened. The first six-ounce beer can was introduced by Schlitz in 1954. Cone-top beer cans were first introduced in 1959. Aluminum beer cans were launched by

Coors in 1960. Between 1960 and 1990, lager started to take over as the country's preferred beer style. That was accomplished by the 1990s. Of the 230 breweries in operation in 1961, 140 were privately held. The year 1962 saw the introduction of the tab-top beer can by the Pittsburgh Brewing Company. Metal kegs were first used in Germany in 1964 (Meussdoerffer, 2009).

Beer cans with "ring pulls" were developed. The first company to sell 10 million barrels in a single year was Budweiser. For the first time ever in the United States, canned beer outsold bottled beer in 1969.

For the first time since before the start of Prohibition in 1920, homebrewing of beer was allowed in the United States in 1978. A home could generate up to 200 gallons tax-free. It could, however, become unlawful in several states and municipalities. The creation of the American Homebrewers Association was a reflection of the rising acceptance of homebrewing. It represented one of the 20th century's most significant movements in beer history.

Colorado hosted the first Great American Beer Festival (GABF) in 1981. It is now the oldest and biggest beer competition and tasting in the country. The nation's first authorized brew pub debuted in 1982. In a brew pub, both food and beer are sold. Since 1920, doing so had been forbidden. The 20th century saw another beer milestone when Budweiser introduced the beer Bud Light.

At the start of 1983, there were 80 breweries run by 51 brewing companies. The six major breweries (Anheuser-Busch, Miller, Heileman, Stroh, Coors, and Pabst) produced 92% of the nation's beer during this time period, marking the lowest point for U.S. breweries in the 20th century.

Asahi Super Dry beer was first made available in Japan in 1989. The Beer Orders were adopted in the UK. Their goal was to eliminate the "tied houses" system used by major breweries. Iceland abolished its almost 80-year-old prohibition on the manufacturing and importing of beer. Twenty percent of the beer produced worldwide in 1991 was made in the United States. In 1992, Finland reinstated and modified the Wife-Carrying Contest. It is based on an ancient custom. Prospective gang members were put to the test by carrying Hefty bags through an obstacle course by Ronkainen the Robber. The champions of the new competition get their wife's weight in beer.

In 1993, Germany modified the 1516 *Reinheitsgebot* legislation to let foreign breweries sell their beer there. The United States legalized the labelling of beer containers with the alcohol content in 1994. In 1995, Interbrew, a Belgian company, acquired Labatt's of Canada. The history of beer in the 20th century has shown significant consolidation. Tutankhamun Ale was produced in 1996. It was brewed using emmer wheat, a primitive variety of the grain, and was a recreation of ancient Egyptian beer.

2.9 21ST CENTURY AND BEER

In 2002, the Miller Brewing Company was purchased by South African Breweries (SAB). In 2004, the largest brewery in Brazil, AmBev, and Interbrew of Belgium united to establish InBev. In 2005, the Finnish brewery Laitilan produced the first beer without gluten. Additionally, it was the first beer to have the worldwide trademark for gluten-free goods.

Anheuser-Busch was purchased by the Belgian brewing firm InBev in 2008. The largest brewery in the world was thus formed. Budweiser declared that Vietnam would now be able to purchase its beer. Carlsberg and Heineken purchased Scottish and Newcastle, the largest breweries in the United Kingdom.

Breweries in Germany were ordered to stop promoting beer as being good for people's health and appearance by a Berlin state court in 2011. The first cassava beer to be manufactured commercially was marketed by SABMiller.

In 2013, more than 25% of the beer brewed worldwide was produced in China. Alabama dropped its threat of legal action against anyone who brewed beer at home. Homebrewing remained prohibited in the dry areas of the state. In Mississippi, homebrewing of beer was now permitted. Homebrewing remained prohibited in the dry areas of the state.

In 2014, England's House of Commons voted to abolish the "beer tie," which dates back 400 years. In this arrangement, bar owners receive cheaper rent in exchange for only purchasing alcohol from their parent firm. In 2015, Anheuser-Busch InBev acquired SABMiller, a close competitor. The merged business has its headquarters in Belgium.

2.10 CRAFT BREWERY REVOLUTION

The 20th century was headed towards a relatively uniform end. Many breweries took the safe route. Pilsner was being brewed in 10,000 different varieties in Germany, and the rest of the globe was doing the same. Many nations were satisfied with only one or two state-owned breweries, and Britain was just beginning to recover from the destruction of its brewing sector due to imports and subpar domestic breweries.

All American beer was tasteless. Then, as a result of the 1980s homebrewing fad, craft beer began to emerge in the United States. This resulted in the revival of forgotten beers like IPAs, sours, and wild-fermented ales. As U.S. craft beer gained popularity, experimentation spread to other nations. For some nations, like Japan, this began early, and it has gradually taken off and expanded to practically every nation: Portugal, Poland, Turkey, Cyprus, and Mexico. Craft beer is revolutionizing the beer landscape worldwide.

2.11 REFERENCES

Cabras, I., & Higgins, D. M. (2016). Beer, brewing, and business history. *Business History, 58*(5), 609–624.

Donnachie, I. (1979). *A history of the brewing industry in Scotland*. John Donald Publishers Ltd.

Hornsey, I. S. (2003). *A history of beer and brewing* (Vol. 34). Royal Society of Chemistry.

Jackowski, M., & Trusek, A. (2018). Non-alcoholic beer production–an overview. *Polish Journal of Chemical Technology, 20*(4).

Meussdoerffer, F. G. (2009). A comprehensive history of beer brewing. In *Handbook of brewing: Processes, technology, markets* (pp. 1–42). Wiley.

Mittelman, A. (2008). *Brewing battles: A history of American beer*. Algora Publishing.

Szymczak, K. (2019). Trade names of beer in Polish: Typology test. *Linguistische Treffen in Wrocław, 16*, 177–190.

3 Fermentation Types and Methods for Brewing

Fermentation is the conversion of "sugars" into alcohol, carbon dioxide, and heat by yeast that leads to the conversion of wort to beer. Sugars are primarily derived from malted barley in most traditional beers, though other cereal sources and plant sugars can also be used. These materials also contribute proteinaceous substances, which, when combined with sugars and flavoring agents such as hops, produce the alcohol, flavors, and aromas that we associate with beer.

In addition, this results in the production of fermentation by-products, which play a vital role in the flavor, aroma, and other characteristics that set beer apart from other beverages. These by-products are formed as a result of the yeast's metabolism, which is the only context in which they can be taken into account. They are partially destroyed as a result of the yeast's metabolism.

The fermentation system itself is made up of a cascading series of three stirred vessels and a fourth unstirred vessel where the beer is separated from the yeast. The system uses a flocculent yeast strain that settles quickly at the end of fermentation. From the fourth vessel, the clarified beer flows to a warm maturation vessel, where the flavor is refined by yeast action from the small amount of residual yeast in the beer. The total residence time in these four vessels can be anything from 40 to 120 hours, depending on production requirements. All different types of beer are produced on the same continuous process line, and their respective differences are produced after the maturation stage (Campbell et al., 2017).

Fermentation and maturation procedures are performed in two ways:

- Many breweries use open formation tanks for fermentation and lagering containers for conditioning. The term "conventional fermentation and maturation" refers to this process.
- In new plants, cylindroconical tanks are used for the fermentation and maturation processes.

3.1 CONVENTIONAL FERMENTATION

Some breweries have open fermentation tanks and lager tanks, and they do the fermentation and maturation in a typical, or classical, manner. The machinery in fermentation and lagering cellars, as well as the fermentation and maturation process, must be taken into account.

Fermentation is carried out in fermentation tanks. Fermentation tanks have different construction materials and use different amounts of area. To get rid of the heat created by fermentation, they are cooled. Construction and lining materials

DOI: 10.1201/b22906-3

for the tanks include wood, steel, aluminum, and concrete with a variety of laminates (pitch, synthetic resins, enamel) utilized as cooling lining for fermentation vessels.

Typically, cooling jackets or, less frequently, cooling coils that flow fresh water cooled to 0–1°C are used to remove heat. The flow of cooling water must be controlled in order to create the proper temperature.

3.2 OPEN TANK FERMENTATION

The fermentation cellar's arrangement of the fermenting tanks makes for effective functioning. It includes a mechanism for removing the carbon dioxide generated by the process, which is chilled.

By pitching the wort, primary fermentation is started. Controlling the temperature and length of the initial fermentation relies on effective fermentation management. Before the beer is sent to the lager cellar, the level of attenuation is assessed. Pitch refers to the act of adding yeast to wort in order to initiate fermentation.

The wort is referred to as pitching wort right before the addition of yeast. Previously, and in certain countries even today, the original wort concentration was indicated in degrees Plato. It is now reported as percent Plato.

The pitched wort is thus already referred to as beer or, rather, as "green young beer," following the yeast addition. When pitching, it is important to provide the yeast enough oxygen access in the wort to start fast multiplication and fermentation as well as to disperse the yeast throughout the wort. This procedure is known as rousing.

The uniform dispersion of the yeast in the wort with the least amount of yeast dumps possible results in the activation (rousing) of the yeast, which happens along with the addition of oxygen. The nutrients in the wort must be quickly contacted by the individual yeast cells. This has an impact on how intense the early fermentation is. As a result, in current plants, the yeast is evenly dosed into the stream of wort that is flowing.

Smaller breweries frequently rouse their yeast by flowing from one vessel to another, by employing a rousing tool, or by utilizing a yeast flask. Modern brewers employ special devices to add tiny air bubbles. Venturi pipes, metal candles, etc. are used for wort aeration.

Poor wort aeration can result in defective early fermentation, a prolonged fermentation period (up to three or more days), and other negative effects like stopping the extraction process, improper secondary fermentation, and issues with beer quality. There is no need to be concerned about too-thorough wort aeration. The yeast eagerly absorbs the oxygen provided here since it needs it so badly to flourish. As a result, oxygen leaves the wort within a few hours and has no negative effects. On the other hand, insufficient yeast aeration is harmful for the reasons outlined earlier.

Now, the yeast is evenly distributed throughout the wort. In order for fermentation to start quickly and strongly, the wort should be forcefully aerated simultaneously.

Between 20 and 30 million yeast cells/hl are added to the wort. The pitching rate has a significant impact on the fermenting period and yeast crop: the higher the pitching rate, the quicker the fermentation period at the same temperature, and the greater the amount of yeast that can be harvested. A pump or valve is used to administer yeast from the yeast buffer tank. A turbidity-monitoring device may be used to regulate the dosage of yeast.

The quantity of yeast cells isn't really counted, of course, but an extrapolation is done, and the rate at which the cells are administered is determined by measuring the turbidity of the wort/yeast solution.

There are several ways to keep track of the yeast addition. It is now extremely common to use turbidity to estimate cell count indirectly. This allows yeast pitching to be automated and may be done in line. A turbidity difference measurement is often employed. For this, the difference in the turbidity of the wort before and after the yeast dose is used to calculate the yeast cell count.

Measuring the yeast load is an alternate technique. Flow rate and solids quantity are combined to provide a measurement parameter (mass per unit volume in g/l) in this case. This approach allows the solids content of a volume to be expressed in kg dry weight by connecting the signals via a process controller. Thus, the consistency of the yeast solution has no bearing on the yeast addition.

The most effective method of faster fermentation without unwanted effects is to increase the yeast addition. The filterability of the beer and the head retention are both positively impacted by an extensive early fermentation.

Typically, yeast is added to the fermenter. After chilling, the yeast still includes some insoluble material that settles to the bottom of the fermenter after about a day. It is made up of hop resins that have re-precipitated after cooling and trub particles that were not captured during trub separation.

Additionally, yeast cells that are weak or dead sink to the bottom. As a result, pitching containers are frequently employed. When a pitching tank is employed, the wort is poured into the tank and emptied after 12 to 24 hours into the fermentation cellar.

Compared to direct pitching in the fermenter, the yeast gathered in the pitching tank is purer and lighter in color. Although 6–7°C is the typical pitching temperature, different temperatures can be employed and often are.

Drauflassen is a specific sort of pitching method (topping up). Topping up refers to adding more wort to a tank that is already fermenting. Fresh wort is added, and the yeast is instantly reactivated, triggering the start of fermentation. The time needed for the initial fermentation stage is shortened by topping up.

However, it is crucial that the wort being added is at the same temperature as the wort that is fermenting when doing this. A shock to the yeast might cause the fermentation to slow down or stop altogether. Temperature variations of any size can have a big impact.

By pitching in line with the rhythm of the wort production cycle, the delayed effects of the induction and acceleration stages are eliminated. This process involves pumping "young beer" from the bottom of a large fermenter, which is filled with deep froth at the high krausen stage. In addition, cooled wort at the same temperature (8.5°C) is delivered from above into the "krausen tank" to maintain a steady level of wort while the young beer ferments further in smaller fermenters. In the krausen tank, the unfermented wart is combined with the young beer that is fermenting, causing the yeast to continue to divide and stay in the yeast multiplication phase.

Theoretically, pitching can continue until there is no more wort available if the amount added is regulated so that the difference between extract in the young beer pumped off and extract in the pitching extract is always 1.5–2.5%. At the same time, the yeast is made up almost entirely of young, sterile cells that ferment quickly. In order to get a significant amount of yeast growth throughout this process, the cold wort must undergo vigorous aeration. There is no reduction in fermentation time if the aeration is insufficient.

The krausen tanks are pumped empty at the end of each week, cleaned, and then refilled with the first brews of the following week and thrown.

The wort is known as green beer as soon as the yeast is added. The green young beer goes through a number of fermentation stages during primary fermentation, and each one is identifiable by its outward manifestation. In managing fermentation, the temperature and duration of the fermentation are crucial factors.

3.3 FERMENTATION STAGES

Initially, the white coating of fine bubble foam covers the green young beer, turning it completely white (or "whitening over" it). Fermentation has started.

Low krausen: There are brown caps on the thin bubble foam. The foam coating should be creamy and appear as homogeneous as possible.

High krausen: The most intensive phase of fermentation, is now underway The foam starts to have greater ridges or crests and coarser bubbles.

Krausen collapsing: Since less carbon dioxide is being produced, the fermentation has become less vigorous, and the high crests are gradually subsiding. The foam appears more brown in color.

Collapsed foam: The pace of fermentation continues to slow down, causing the foam to collapse until it eventually reduces to a thin, soiled brown coating that must be removed before transferring the beer to prevent it from sinking and killing the yeast.

3.4 FERMENTATION TEMPERATURE

The pitching temperature and the maximum temperature are significant in terms of temperature management during bottom primary fermentation. The green young beer has to be chilled again to pitching temperature once primary fermentation is complete. Normal pitching temperatures range from 5 to 6°C. The pitching temperature is typically increased in shorter procedures to kick-start the fermentation more rapidly.

The temperature of the wort rises as a result of the heat emitted during fermentation. Although fermentation moves along more rapidly at higher temperatures, considerable care is required to not go over a set maximum temperature for quality reasons. Cold fermentation, which has a maximum temperature of 8 to 9°C, and warm fermentation, which has a maximum temperature of 10 to 15°C, are distinguished based on this minimum temperature.

For one to two days, the maximum temperature is kept as steady as possible. The young green beer is then gradually chilled. Because yeast is sensitive to significant temperature decreases, the temperature should be reduced gradually and steadily, not more than 1 K every day. At transfer, the temperature is around 4–5°C (Willaert, 2005).

Temperature, extract content, and pH values for many significant parameters change during the fermentation process. It is crucial for the person in charge of the fermentation to keep an eye on and regulate the temperature throughout primary fermentation and, more importantly, to quantify the extraction loss during the primary fermentation's last days. Typically, main fermentation takes six to eight days.

3.5 DEGREE OF ATTENUATION

The extract is continuously fermented throughout fermentation. *Vergarungsgrad* (V), or "degree of fermentation," refers to the degree of conversion to alcohol. How much of the extract in the pitching wort has been fermented can be determined by the degree of attenuation.

The difference between the extract content of the pitching wort and that of the beer at any particular time is called the fermented extract. The percentage attenuation (V) is calculated from the equation:

$$V\ (\%) = (\text{fermented extract/extract in the pitching wort}) * 100$$

3.6 APPARENT ATTENUATION (V_s)

A hydrometer is used in the fermentation cellar to measure the extract content. However, since the extract value the hydrometer indicates (AE) is incorrect due to the produced alcohol, the attenuation measured with the hydrometer is only ostensibly right (V). However, since AE can be measured readily and there is a proportionate link between the higher inaccuracy and increasing attenuation, the apparent attenuation is always employed in practice.

3.7 REAL ATTENUATION

In the lab, the alcohol needs to be distilled out and replaces with water to get the true percentage of attenuation. This number is used in the computation to get the actual percentage attenuation (V_w). Real attenuation always decreases more slowly than perceived attenuation.

$$V_w \approx V_s * 0.81$$

3.8 CYLINDROCONICAL TANKS (CCVs)

Up to a certain size, the formerly common fermenters and storage tanks can be utilized. Larger production facilities for the fermentation and ageing of beer were eventually introduced in response to the desire for greater profitability and higher volume. The cylindroconical fermentation and lagering containers, which the majority of breweries today deem essential, have produced fully successful outcomes. They not only offer operational benefits but also guarantee that the beer's quality is preserved during fermentation and maturing.

Cylindrical tanks can be built up to 40 meters high and more than 10 meters in diameter. As a consequence of experience and testing, which demonstrate it is preferable not to exceed specific predetermined measures, there is currently a little bit more attention paid to determining the dimensions, especially in the case of cylindrical fermentation containers.

Tests have revealed that wort height has an impact on the characteristics of the by-products of fermentation. A 20 m CO_2-containing wort column is exerting pressure on a yeast cell that is fermenting at that depth. Thus, the CO_2 content sets a ceiling on the height of the wort column that can be generated. The maximum wort height in a cylindrical fermenter should be 20 m in light of current understanding. However, there are many cylindrical fermentation containers with a 23–27 m fill height. In a cylindrical lagering tank, wort height is irrelevant as long as diacetyl removal has completed the maturing process.

The ideal diameter-to–wort height ratio in cylindrical fermentation tanks is a subject of debate. From 1:1 to 1:5, the ratio changes. Wider vessels have recently received greater attention; the diameter-to-total wort height ratio should be 1:2, and the diameter-to-cylindrical wort height ratio should be 1.4:1.5. The diameter-to-height ratio affects the homogeneity of the content in CCVs with cooling jackets, particularly when only a tiny quantity of CO_2 is produced.

The majority of tanks have diameters between 3.50 and 4.50 m, which make them challenging to carry. Cone angles typically range from 60 to 75 degrees but can reach 90 degrees. For computations, it's crucial to understand that a cone with a 60° angle has a height equal to the diameter times 0.866.

It goes without saying that the cylindrical fermentation containers cannot be totally filled for fermentation since, in these vessels as well, the CO_2 evolution produces relatively significant volumes of foam that, in extreme circumstances, can erupt from the gas pipes and stick the safety valves. This poses a serious risk since the adhering wort may completely obstruct the valves, rendering them inoperable. In essence, this means that the headspace volume in fermentation tanks should be equivalent to 18 to 25% of the volume of pitched wort.

3.9 FERMENTATION IN CYLINDROCONICAL TANKS

Nowadays, fermentation and maturation are carried out in cylindrical vessels wherever possible, but due to the wide variety of technical equipment in breweries and accepted practices, it is also possible to utilize a combination of traditional fermentation and lagering vessels and CCVs.

The yeast is immediately added to the wort at a concentration of 20 to 30 million yeast cells per mL (20 to $30*10^6$ yeast cells/m1); as the wort ferments, the cell concentration rises to 60 to 80 million yeast cells per mL. The number of cells present during pitching affects the rate of fermentation and other biochemical processes. If the temperature is maintained, increasing the pitching causes the fermentation to be more intense, the yeast to grow less, the maximum concentration of vicinal diketones to increase and occur earlier, the removal of green beer aromas to occur more quickly, the reduction of mature beer aromas to occur more slowly, the loss of bitter substances during primary fermentation at atmospheric pressure to increase, and the danger to the autolysis to increase.

When yeast cells are pitched, ageing markers also rise along with them; as a result, the flavor stability declines as the pitching rate rises. In the event of cold fermentation, the pitching temperature is 8–10°C, while in the case of warm fermentation, it is 14–18°C. To avoid shocking the yeast, the wort that is coming in must be at the same temperature as the batch that has previously been pitched.

The effects of raising the pitching temperature include accelerated yeast growth, intensified yeast metabolism, increased turbulence and better yeast distribution, a quicker and lower pH drop, increased excretion of nitrogenous and bitter substances, an increase in alcohol content and an unfavorable alcohol-to-esters ratio, less aromatic and emptier beers, a decrease in volatile acids, and an increase in fixed acids.

From a microbiological perspective, pitching must commence at the beginning of the wort input and be dispersed throughout the entire volume. Therefore, it is necessary to incorporate the yeast dose and aeration devices into the wort flow. Without yeast, wort bacteria that are created from spores, which multiply ten times more quickly than yeast, can thrive within a matter of hours and rob the wort of essential vitamins and growth agents. Pitching can be done with harvested yeast alone, with harvested yeast and propagated yeast mixed together, or by krausening after topping up.

A mixture of 70% harvested yeast and 30% propagated yeast is frequently preferred due to the faster fermentation with a uniform high quality, higher SO_2 content, lower investment costs, smaller amounts of surplus yeast, and better yeast clarification that can be anticipated, despite the additional work and increased microbiological risk (Debourg, 2010).

According to general norms, the aerated cast wort should have an oxygen concentration of 5.5 to 8.0 mg/L (12%) at a maximum oxygen saturation of 60 to 80% with air; 4.5 to 6 mg O_2/L wort is required for CCVs to ferment and mature more quickly. Increased aeration causes more yeast to grow, more intense fermentation, less nitrogen in the finished beet, a faster pH drop, more acetaldehyde and vicinal diketone precursors to form, more esters and higher alcohols to form during the fermentation stage, more bitter substances to be lost during primary fermentation, and less hydrogen sulfide and DMS to form.

Severe rates of aeration result in excessive wort oxidation, an increased risk of ageing, expensive processes and energy usage, strong foam creation, inefficient space utilization, excessive foam substance loss, and oxidative stress for the yeast cells.

According to an outdated brewing regulation, fermentation and lagering should last one week each for every percentage of original extract content. This adage no longer holds true, and even half the lagering period is typically not permitted.

For a brewery to be profitable, the beer needs to ferment and develop in the shortest amount of time. Today, fermentation, maturation, and lagering can often be completed in 17 to 20 days, and there is a trend to cut these times even more while retaining the same level of quality.

This is also conceivable with conventional fermentation and maturation, but fermentation and maturation in ceramic vessels also offer excellent options for process modification while preserving high quality.

Particular attention must be paid to a few factors while fermenting and maturing in cylindrical tanks in less than three weeks, especially as it is no longer possible to acquire a visual idea of how the fermentation is progressing during this period.

First and foremost, level of nitrogen compounds is crucial in the wort produced during the mashing. It is ideal for wort to have 23 mg FAN per 100 mL or more, since this will guarantee that the yeast is receiving the right nutrients. When adjuncts are employed, the FAN level of all malt wort must be at least 15 mg/100 mL and cannot be less than 20 mg/100 mL.

As was already discussed, wort aeration and yeast pitching rate are crucial components for a quick and active start to fermentation. Approximately one liter of thick yeast slurry per hl is produced by pitching yeast at a rate of 30 million yeast cells per mL.

Aeration at regular intervals during the start phase ensures that the yeast gets the oxygen supply it needs to grow; however, persistent aeration of 2 m^3 air/h during the start phase causes the beer to oxidize excessively and negatively. Instead of "a lot helps a lot," the start-phase mantra should be "aeration at intervals." Additionally, it should be noted that the yeast already transitions from the logarithmic phase to the delayed phase at alcohol concentrations of 0.7–0.8% and from the delayed phase to the stationary phase at 1.5%. However, air is necessary, even in modest amounts, as long as development is occurring.

The most detrimental element for flavor stability is oxygen. However, aeration is thought to be essential while pitching since, in the absence of aeration, yeast growth is thought to be minimal or nonexistent, and fermentation duration rises. Whether all brews must be aerated or only part of them is of utmost importance. The flavor and flavor stability of the beer are improved as a result of the yeast producing SO_2. While only created near the conclusion of fermentation, SO_2 is a by-product of the production of amino acids containing sulfur. However, when aeration is at its lowest, SO_2 production is at its highest. Aeration should be halted to prevent SO_2 production at an alcohol level exceeding 1.5%. In order to retain fermentation activity and to have a positive impact on SO_2 generation and, in turn, the flavor and ageing stability of the beer, it is advisable to minimize or cease aerating the final brews.

High-vitality yeast does not produce any SO_2, and only after a yeast cycle does it become significantly more capable of doing so. When pitching, a mixture of collected yeast (60%) and assimilation yeast (40%) should be utilized to produce a high SO_2 level in a reasonable amount of time.

Using an aerobic yeast cycle, modern yeast management keeps yeasts in their best physiological state. These yeasts may ferment in completely non-aerated worts because they received enough oxygen during culture, preventing the introduction of oxygen, which has a negative impact on the acceptability of ageing. In any event, the initial brew should be the sole time the wort is aerated; otherwise, all subsequent brews should be aerated less vigorously.

Due to its sensitivity to abrupt temperature fluctuations and shock symptoms from abrupt chilling, yeast has negative effects on fermentation and cell division. Rapid cooling must always be avoided during the initial and logarithmic phases, and if topping off is done, the extra wort should be at the same temperature as the original batch.

Diacetyl elimination is a sign of how well a beer is maturing. The other green beer scents should also be gone if practically all the diacetyl has been eliminated. At the conclusion of maturation, the "total diacetyl" concentration (vicinal diketones) should be less than 0.1 mg/L. During lagering, a minor quantity is also taken out. Beer should have a diacetyl content of less than 0.10 mg/L, and any yeast that has been added should be withdrawn from the tank as soon as the consistency permits. Autolyzed yeast degrades the flavor of beer.

All beers should be chilled to between 1 and 2°C after maturity and held there for at least seven days to obtain the necessary colloidal stability. If no external cooler is utilized, cooling generally takes around 70 hours. More money must be spent on stabilization since lagering times are shorter and lagering temperatures are higher.

The maximum fermentation temperature ranges from 10–12°C under cold fermentation circumstances to 14–16°C under warm fermentation conditions to 1–2°C higher in the maturation phase.

An increase in temperature during the fermentation stage results in an increase in yeast propagation (higher extract loss); an increase in fermentation activity (shorter fermentation phase); an increase in formation of higher alcohols, esters, aldehydes, and vicinal diketones; an increase in DMS and lower H_2S concentrations; a faster fall in pH value; and lower pH in the final product. Temperature and pressure are the two controlling variables that determine these results.

An increase in temperature during the maturation stage speeds up the conversion of the diacetyl and the reduction of other green beer aroma compounds, which accelerates maturation. It also increases the risk of yeast autolysis, lowers the content of soluble CO_2, and increases the likelihood that excreted components will dissolve again.

An increase in pressure during fermentation results in a decrease in yeast growth, a decrease in fermentation activity and a longer fermentation phase, a decrease in the formation of intermediate products of fermentation, a slower pH decline and a higher beer pH, a decrease in the loss of bitter substances, a decrease in protein excretion, a decrease in turbulence as a result of a decrease in CO release, and an increase in the CO_2 content in the finished beer.

An increase in average temperature of 1°C is countered by a 0.16 bar rise in bunging pressure. It should be noted that during primary fermentation, green beer should only be chilled by a maximum of 1–1.5°C every day. Otherwise, there is a risk of shocking the yeast, which can significantly reduce yeast growth and cause damage to the yeast batch. In the worst situation, fermentation may stop.

Additionally, the mobility of the substrate that is fermenting might affect fermentation: Increased movement during the fermentation stage results in increased yeast growth, increased fermentation intensity, increased and faster pH value decline, increased bitter substance loss, more intense protein excretion, decreased head retention, increased formation of green beer aroma substances, increased formation of mature beer aroma substances, and decreased free fatty acid levels (Annemuller et al., 2004).

Increased movement during the maturation stage has several negative effects, including driving the maturation reactions owing to more quickly broken down processes, a more rapid dispersion of yeast excretion compounds in the beer, and a higher danger of CO_2 losses.

The use of a green beer separator, clarification aids (no longer used in Germany), sudden and rapid cooling of the tank's contents, a rapid increase in pressure at the end of the fermentation phase to 0.8–1.0 bar, and yeast with a clearly flocculent character all work to hasten yeast sedimentation.

3.10 METHODS OF FERMENTATION

Cold lagering can be executed either in a cylindroconical lagering vessel and fermentation in a cylindroconical fermentation vessel—a two-tank process—or both processes can be performed in a single CCV. Hence, CCVs can serve a dual purpose.

The fermentation can likewise be carried out in a cylindrical vessel, and the maturation and lagering can be done in standard lagering tanks. To ensure consistent beer quality while using the two-tank method, maturing (diacetyl removal) must be carried out in the cylindrical fermentation vessel. Therefore, only cold lagering for colloidal stabilization, clarity, and flavor muffling should be done in the cylindrical lagering vessel.

Basically, the one-tank method offers the following significant benefits:

> There are fewer cleaning expenses because only one vessel needs to be cleaned, fewer CO_2 losses because one does not transfer under pressure to an empty tank, fewer beer losses because there are no pipe losses or wetting losses, fewer labor hours required because there is no beer transfer, fewer energy costs because the beer is not pumped over, and fewer risks associated with oxygen intake (Moerman et al., 2014).

Because foam headspace is no longer needed, the vessel volume utilization is poorer during the lagering stage. The two methods do not fundamentally produce beer of different quality. Practically every fermentation procedure can be carried out in a single tank or two.

Recovery of CO_2 is always required or highly recommended for fiscal and environmental reasons. Only warm maturing procedures and low pressures require carbonation. For each tank, a cooling system is a fundamental need.

There are three categories of cold fermentation: cold maturation and cold fermentation, warm maturation, and warm fermentation, and cold maturation that can be used to categorize the fermentation and maturing processes for bottom-fermentation beers.

3.11 COLD MATURATION AND COLD FERMENTATION

Regarding customary fermentation and maturation, this procedure has previously been discussed. When pitching, the temperature is kept between 6–7°C and allowed to increase to 8–9°C. The peak temperature is attained after about two days, and it is maintained for another two days before gradually dropping to 3–4°C. The beer is then transferred while still holding residual fermentable extract, with the difference between it and the attenuation limit being between 1.1 and 1.3% in the case of open tank fermentation and 0.8 to a maximum of 1.0% when utilizing a CCV.

Then, it is carefully chilled to lagering temperature so that the yeast can reduce any remaining diacetyl to a level below the cutoff (0.1 mg/L). After that, the beer is aged for at least another week at –1°C. More than five weeks of extended lagering is not advised. Processes in lager cellars must constantly be carefully monitored. If this isn't done, the beer may taste yeasty; start to autolyze with an increase in pH; or have flavor, froth, and stability issues, among other things.

Transfer using krausen is a unique procedure. The addition of green young beer at the low krausen (low foam) stage, when the attenuation is around 25%, is referred to as krausening. When there is not enough extract left in the beer, krausening is frequently used to produce extract for secondary fermentation. However, this is an emergency solution; thus it is not the topic here. The fact that many brewers purposefully add krausen upon transfer to enhance the froth and flavor is what makes this situation interesting. The beer is virtually entirely fermented for this purpose in a robust primary fermentation, and this beer is transferred at about 10–12% krausen at around 5°C without the now sufficiently sedimented primary fermentation yeast. Krausening makes high-quality beer, but in order to prevent the primary fermentation yeast from tainting the beer, it must be cleaned as thoroughly as possible.

3.12 COLD FERMENTATION WITH ACCELERATED MATURATION

This technique involves pitching at 6–7°C and allowing the temperature to increase to 8–9°C. However, in this process, the beer is transported to the cylindrical tank at the same temperature while the maximum temperature is maintained. Krausen, or green young beer with little froth, is added to the green beer at a rate of around 10% during transfer. As a result, the active yeast in the beer is fermenting, significantly lowering the quantity of diacetyl that is still present to below the threshold level. It is not chilled until this point; instead, it is stored at a lagering temperature of –1°C for a week.

Yeast must be eliminated every two to four days after the final attenuation is obtained, which should be as near as possible to the attenuation limit, with the last removal occurring naturally before filtering. A 20-day production cycle is typical.

3.13 COLD MATURATION—WARM FERMENTATION WITHOUT PRESSURE

The fact that all fermentation and maturation processes move more quickly at higher temperatures is taken advantage of in the quest to speed up these processes. As a result, substantially more diacetyl is produced when pitching is done at 8°C and the temperature is allowed to increase to 12–14°C, but it is also eliminated more quickly and thoroughly.

The beer is not chilled to the lagering temperature of –1°C, and the cold lagering phase is maintained for a week until the diacetyl is removed. The procedure can also be carried out in a typical basement and lasts for 17 to 20 days.

The procedure has the following benefits: ultimate attenuation is obtained extremely fast, diacetyl is swiftly and consistently eliminated, high-quality beer is produced, and the process has also been successfully used in pressure fermentation.

3.14 WITH-PRESSURE FERMENTATION

Naturally, more fermentation by-products occur if the temperature is allowed to increase even more: for example, over 20°C. Unless pressure limits the synthesis of more diacetyl and other by-products, this continues without interruption. Of course, this requires that pressure vessels approved for operation at the requisite pressure are readily accessible.

The applied pressure is increased to the estimated desired counterpressure at an attenuation of around 50%. This pressure is kept constant until the maturation period is complete, at which point it is decreased to the counterpressure necessary for lagering. On the ninth or tenth day of chilling, a cold lagering phase at –1°C is once more used for at least a week. It takes this process between 17 and 20 days.

3.15 WARM MATURATION—COLD FERMENTATION

A lot of fermentation by-products are always produced during warm fermentation. The benefit of cold fermentation and warm maturation is that fewer by-products are produced, and these by-products may readily be eliminated during warmer maturation.

When using a cold primary fermentation with integrated maturation, the fermentation is carried out at 8–9°C until the fermenter has attenuated by about 50%, at which point cooling is turned off, and the temperature increases to 12–13°C on its own. The beer is moved and lagered cold for a week after a maturation phase in which the diacetyl removal is under control, or it is chilled in the tank to –1°C and lagered (one-tank process). Without carbonation, a CO_2 concentration of 5.4–5.6 g/l can be attained with one bar of overpressure. A typical lager cellar can also be used to carry out this operation. About 20 days are needed to complete the process.

3.16 WARM FERMENTATION—COLD MATURATION

The ability to significantly reduce fermentation time by raising temperature has been demonstrated. The amount of fermentation by-products increases, the beer tends to develop yeasty-floral fragrance notes with rising temperature, and foam and colloidal stability are often worse as a result.

The fermentation process may be shortened to four days, which significantly increases capacity. Only warm fermentation, krausening, and the utilization of particular maturation conditions are often practical (Annemuller & Manger, 2005).

3.17 YEAST CROPPING

During yeast cropping, the yeast is initially transported from the tank cone to an expansion tank while under pressure. Because the CO_2, which is deadly to the yeast, is immediately released, the yeast is still foaming vigorously there. The yeast is given oxygen at the same time for two to three hours. Now, the yeast can either be used again immediately for pitching, or it can be used again after potential treatment and cold storage.

It is important to gather the yeast often and as early as feasible. This is due to a number of factors. The yeast does not settle as desired. Up to the conclusion of the maturation stage, higher cell densities on the surface occur following the turbulence of the primary fermentation, which is brought on by active yeast cells rising. There are also ebullitions of yeast clouds from the heated sediment in the cone during cold lagering. However, the majority of the yeast eventually settles in the cone, with the sedimentation period being significantly influenced by the height of the tank. As quickly as possible, the yeast that has already settled should be removed (Cheong et al., 2007).

In particular, low-molecular-weight proteins that can no longer be absorbed by the body of the beer are excreted by the yeast, which has a detrimental impact on head retention. The yeast excretes proteinase A as the beer matures and becomes colder, which causes the beer's froth to significantly deteriorate as foam-producing ingredients break down. This is especially crucial for beers that don't receive any heat treatment before filling and that include proteinase A in the end product. Early-collected yeast has a lower capacity to release proteinase than later-collected yeast, while suspended yeast has a lower capacity than sedimented yeast. Hence, early yeast collection yields superior beer quality.

Autolysis products produced by unhealthy yeast have a detrimental impact on the progression of fermentation. The complexes made of protein, glycogen, and mannan dissolve once more and cause turbidity and filtration issues if they exceed the taste threshold (Cheong et al., 2008).

The CO_2 partial pressure, which also enhances this cell toxin in the yeast cells, causes the yeast to suffer, especially in high tanks in the cone. Compared to CO_2, the yeast cell can endure pressure better. The yeast weakens more while it remains in the cone, and as a result, the great cell density in this area scarcely transmits any more nutrients. When their reserve ingredients run out, particularly aged yeast cells (with many bud scars) begin to metabolize their own cell components. Autolysis is the term for this disorder. In this process, the cell's internal and external membranes are broken down by inner secretory enzymes, allowing amino acids, fatty acids, and enzymes—most notably proteinase A—to be expelled. The yeast cell dies as a result of the entire metabolism getting out of control. The substances released have a very negative impact on the quality: through the release of amino acids and proteolytic enzymes, the flavor and foam stability are permanently damaged; the released fatty acids, especially the unsaturated acids, have a negative impact on the flavor stability of the beer; the excreted substances are a culture medium for potential contaminants in the beer; the pH of the beer increases; this is an unmistakable sign that autolysis has occurred.

The percentage of dead cells should be as low as feasible, often between 1 and 2%, and clearly identifiable by methylene blue coloring under a microscope. If the percentage of dead cells keeps rising, there is a risk that more autolysis by-products, notably the proteinase A that reduces foam, may enter the beer.

3.18 REFERENCES

Annemuller, G., & Manger, H. (2005). *Brforum, 6–7*, S15–S148. https://scholar.google.com/scholar?hl=en&as_sdt=0%2C5&q=Annemuller%2C+G.%2C+%26+Manger%2C+H.+%282005%29.+Brforum%2C&btnG=

Annemuller, G., Manger, H. J., & Lietz, P. (2004). *Die Hefe in der Brauerei*. https://www.vlb-berlin.org/sites/default/files/2018-02/Hefe2014-inhalt.pdf

Campbell, C., Nanjundaswamy, A. K., Njiti, V., Xia, Q., & Chukwuma, F. (2017). Value-added probiotic development by high-solid fermentation of sweet potato with Saccharomyces boulardii. *Food science & nutrition*, 5(3), 633–638.

Cheong, C., Wackerbauer, K., Beckmann, M., & Kang, S. A. (2007). Influence of preserved brewing yeast strains on fermentation behavior and flocculation capacity. *Nutrition Research and Practice*, *1*(4), 260–265.

Cheong, C., Wackerbauer, K., Lee, S. K., & Kang, S. A. (2008). Optimal conditions for propagation in bottom and top brewing yeast strains. *Food Science and Biotechnology*, *17*(4), 739–744.

Debourg, A. (2010). Yeast management and high gravity fermentation. *Cerevisia*, *35*(1), 16–22.

Moerman, F., Rizoulières, P., & Majoor, F. A. (2014). Cleaning in place (CIP) in food processing. In *Hygiene in food processing* (pp. 305–383). Woodhead Publishing.

Willaert, R. (2005). Biochemistry and fermentation of beer. In *Handbook of food science, technology, and engineering* (pp. 2993–3012). CRC Press.

4 Raw Material for Beer Manufacturing

4.1 INTRODUCTION

Beer is made of four raw materials: malts (processed barley), water, hops, and yeast. The quality of final product (beer) depends on the quality of these four. Barley is the main raw material used for beer. Hops gives a unique bitter taste to beer. Water is the most important raw material, quantitatively. Its quality plays a great role in final product's quality. Yeast is used for alcoholic fermentation to produce beer (Bamforth, 2006).

4.2 BARLEY

The main cereal utilized as a source of carbohydrates for making beer is barley. Its scientific name is *Hordeum vulgare*, a monocotyledonous grass of the Gramineae family that was first discovered in the Fertile Crescent of the Middle East (formerly Mesopotamia and its surroundings, now Syria, Iraq, and neighboring lands). There is also *H. vulgare spontaneum*, wild barley. It is speculative how ancient civilizations learned how to transform the plant's starch into sugars that could later be fermented to a tasty beverage. The plant was used as a cereal for bread making many thousands of years ago.

Starch present in barley is converted into fermentable or simpler sugars in the brewhouse during mashing. Varieties that provide high extra are cultivated for brewing. Barley is a grain whose ears are distinguished by unusually lengthy awns.

The two main types of barley are the winter barleys, whose seeds are planted in the middle of September, and spring barleys, which are planted in March and April. Both kinds are further separated into varieties as two-row and multi-row (six-row), depending on how the corns are arranged on the ear axis (rachis). There are three fertile florets at each node on the rachis of multi-row barleys (Kunze, 2004).

Large, plump grains with typically thinner, finely wrinkled husks are produced by two-row barleys. Because they include less husk and a greater proportion of useful components, these barleys also have fewer bitter and polyphenolic compounds. The extract content is rather high, and the grains are all fairly uniform. Two-row barleys are best produced as spring barleys since they have all the qualities needed to produce malt and beer.

On the other hand, uneven-size grains are produced by six-row barleys. The grains in the rows from the lateral florets are thinner and crumpled at the distal end where the awns are joined because they do not have enough space to expand completely (twisted grains). Six-row barleys may be identified by their twisted grains.

DOI: 10.1201/b22906-4

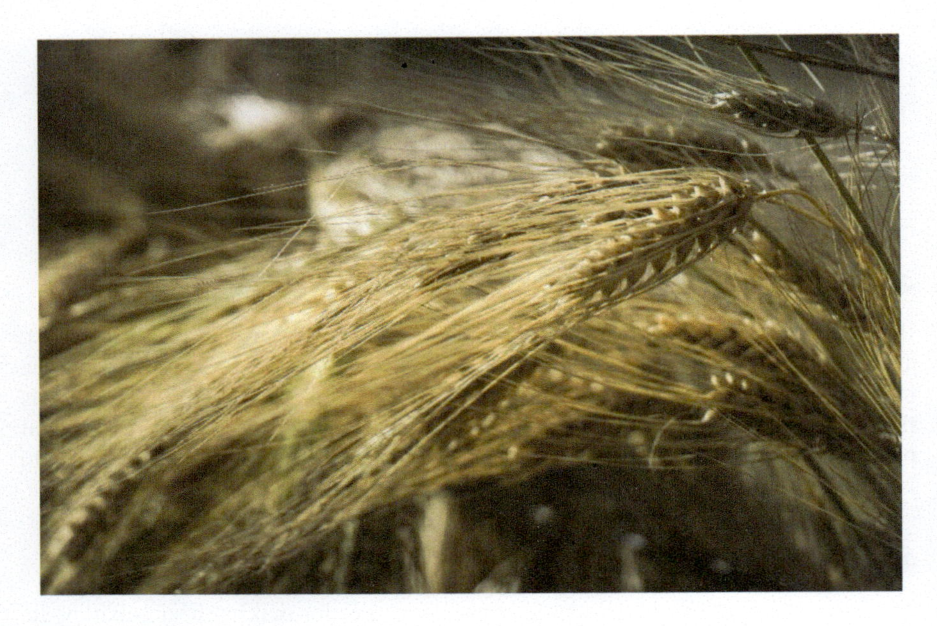

FIGURE 4.1 Barley

About 300 spring barleys, 100 two-row winter barleys, and 100 six-row winter barleys are registered in the European Brewery Convention (EBC) nations alone. Due to deliberate efforts undertaken to enhance their brewing quality for more than a century, two-row spring barleys are by far the best for malting and brewing purposes. Numerous variants have outstanding technical attributes. However, increasing numbers of two-row winter barleys are being developed whose quality is almost as good as that of two-row spring barleys.

Central Europe, where barley has been regularly farmed for nearly 150 years, is where it is most often cultivated. Important varieties include Scarlet, Barke, Pasadena, and Annabel in Germany; Optic and Alliot in Denmark; Chariot and Riviera in Britain; and Astoria and Aspen in France. The breeding of brewing barley is, however, under constant development, so new varieties with improved properties are always coming to the fore (Kunze, 2004).

4.3 STRUCTURE OF THE BARLEY KERNEL

4.3.1 External

The dorsal side of the kernel, which includes the dorsal husk or lemma, is lengthened in the ear of our domesticated barleys by a long awn that is severed during threshing. The lemma's wrinkles serve as a gauge for the husk's fineness, allowing one to assess the husk's tensile strength. The rachilla, the remnants of an infertile floret, and the ventral husk, also known as the palea, are located in the ventral furrow of the kernel and can also be used to identify the variety.

The sort of barley used in the brewing is always husked. In other words, during growing, the ventral and dorsal husks remain closely linked to the pericarp and testa, and they are still present on the kernel after thrashing. The kernel's base has a sharper point than the tip. This makes sense if you keep in mind that during threshing, the awn is stuck off.

4.3.2 Internal

The germ area, the endosperm, and the grain coverings make up the three primary components of the barley kernel. The embryo has growth nodes for the acrospire and rootlets, present in the germ area. The scutellum, a thin layer of palisade-like cells with extremely thin walls, and the epithelium, a thin tissue layer, are what separate the germ area from the endosperm. Starch granules are found in the stable cells that make up the endosperm. The granules of stored starch are both large and small; medium-size granules are absent in the case of barley starch. The diameter of the large granules ranges from 20 to 30 mm, whereas the small granules, with a diameter of 3 to 5 mm, make up 70 to 95% of the endosperm starch granules but only comprise 3 to 10% of the total weight of the starch (Kunze, 2004).

The type of barley and the growth conditions have a significant impact on the quantity of small starch granules. The malting characteristics of the barley and the quality of the malt are also influenced by the small starch granules. An endosperm matrix containing protein fills the space between starch granules, and this matrix component can either be highly dense or completely absent (Schwarz & Li, 2011).

First and foremost, phospholipids and proteins make up the middle lamella of cell walls, which controls all internal and external mass transport. The β-glycan layer is present on both sides of the middle lamella. The diverse compounds, such as organic acids like acetic acid or ferulic acid, are then held in this layer, which is, in turn, coated on both sides by an extremely porous pentosan layer.

The properties of the variety and the growth conditions have a significant impact on the thickness of the starch cell walls. Cell walls of brewing barleys are typically thinner than those of feed barleys. The malting qualities of the barley are significantly influenced by the thickness of the cell walls since thick walls present more obstacles (Gupta et al., 2010).

The aleurone layer, which is made up of cells rich in protein, is located around the endosperm. The generation of enzymes during malting has its most crucial beginning point in this layer. The stable protein structure of this layer is where additional elements, including lipids, polyphenols, and coloring agents, are deposited.

The seven various layers that make up the grain covers may, however, be roughly split into three. The seed coat, or testa, is the outermost covering that surrounds the aleurone layer. It encircles the entire head of the corn and lets only clear water pass through, not the salts dissolved in it. This is caused by the testa's semi-permeability (Kunze, 2004).

The fruit coat, also known as the pericarp, which has evolved very similarly to the seed coat, is the next layer that is found outside. It is encircled by the testa, which is then encircled by the epidermis, which is externally shielded by the two husks of the kernel.

The husks are mostly made of cellulose, but they also contain trace quantities of testinic acid, polyphenols, and bitter compounds that can have a negative impact on the quality of the beer.

4.4 COMPOSITION OF THE COMPONENTS

Barley typically has 13 to 15% moisture. In extremely dry harvesting circumstances, the moisture content can range from 12% to over 20%, whereas in wet conditions, it can reach over 20%. Very wet barley has to be dried since it cannot be kept for an extended period of time and would rapidly lose its potential to germinate. For long-term preservation, barley must have a moisture level below 15%. "Dry matter" is the term used to describe the residual material (Kunze, 2004).

Although carbohydrates are the most significant class of compounds in terms of quantity, they differ greatly from one another in terms of their qualities, which affect how crucial they are for processing and the quality of the final product. Glucose is the simplest kind of sugar. With the help of sunlight as the energy source, glucose is formed from CO_2 and H_2O during the photosynthesis of foliage plants. It is then stored in polymer form as cellulose in higher shrubs or stems or as phase transition material in cereal grains and fruits. The most significant glucose polymers are cellulose and starch (Gupta et al., 2010). Foliage plants create roughly 100 billion tons of these compounds each year through photosynthesis.

4.5 STARCH

The most significant component, starch ($C_6H_{10}O_5$), accounts for 63% of the dry matter in barley. The developing starch grains, which resemble onion peels, are used to store the glucose produced during photosynthesis after it has been carried upward in the stem and polymerized in the grain and mature grain. The size and form of the starch granules in the different types of grain vary greatly. Up to 98% of the starch granules (amyloplasts) are made up of pure starch; the remaining material is made up of proteins, fats, and minerals. There is a distinction between amylose and amylopectin. Barley starch contains between 16 and 24% amylose; small granules can have up to 40% amylose. The granule's inside is where the amylose is concentrated. It has up to 2,000 spirally twisted glucose molecules and is made up of long, unbranched helical chains with a 1,4 linkage (a so-called helix spiral). Through an iodine tincture, chains with more than 8 glucose-retained molecules initially appear red in color, changing to blue as they lengthen (Kunze, 2004).

The majority of the starch granule is made up of amylopectin, which accounts for roughly 80% (76–84%). The amylopectin molecules are branched because, in addition to the 1,4 bond, 1,6 bonds also take place. About ten times bigger than amylose molecules, amylopectin molecules can contain up to 40,000 glucose molecules. Amylopectin molecules resemble a branching tree, with multiple clusters of upright spirals of glucose molecules (double helix with 1,6 bond, around 9 nm long) sprouting from the trunk. Thus, it is conceivable to estimate that in the case of amylopectin, 1,6 bonds make up roughly 6–7% of all bonds. α-glucans are substances like amylose and amylopectin that contain α-glucose. For the brewer, starch is a viable extract source from which to obtain the necessary alcohol (Bamforth, 2006).

4.6 CELLULOSE

Around 5 to 6% of the dry matter in barley is made up of cellulose, which serves as a structural component and is predominantly found in the husk. A β-glucan called cellulose has lengthy chains of 1,4-bonded glucose molecules, making it insoluble and indigestible to humans. Additionally, it is particularly resistant to the effects of enzymes. Later, cellulose exits the manufacturing process unchanged, with its primary usage as a filter material during lautering in the brewhouse. If ingredients held in the husk—such as silica, tannins, and bittering acid—are significantly lixiviated during lautering, the resulting beer may suffer (Kok et al., 2019).

4.7 HEMICELLULOSE

Hemicelluloses are the main constituents of the endosperm cell walls. They consist of glucans and pentosans (polymers of pentoses), which together form the rigid framework of the endosperm cell walls; p-glucans and pentosans have different structures and very different effects on beer production and quality, so they will be considered separately. Hemicelluloses consist of 80 to 90% β-glucan and 10 to 12% pentosan (Gupta et al., 2010).

4.8 β-GLUCANS

Long chains of glucose molecules connected by 1,3 and, more frequently, 1,4 bonds make up β-glucans. β-Glucans are strongly correlated with higher molecular protein molecules and pentosans, and are present in barley and the endosperm cell walls in concentrations of 4 to 7%. When β-glucan is dissolved, hydrogen bonds between the molecules cause them to interact with one another, creating what are known as fringed micelles. During the malting process, the breakdown of β-glucan assumes considerable significance. The final beer may suffer if β-glucan is not broken down enough. Although linked to cellulose, β-glucan is not the same as it can be broken down by enzymes, but, as we will see, this has to happen in the maltings because mashing can only partially correct it (Kunze, 2004).

4.9 PENTOSANS

The pentoses xylose and arabinose make up the majority of pentosans, which are polymers of pentoses. Pentosans are essentially made up of long chains of 1,4-D-xylose residues, to which arabinose residues are sometimes attached via 1,2 or 1,3 bonds. About 67% of the aleurone layer, 50% of the shell, and 20% of the endosperm are composed of pentosans. Pentosans are also degraded enzymatically, although the rate of decomposition is very low (only 11–20%), leaving a significant amount of high-molecular pentosans behind at the conclusion of malting.

4.10 PROTEINS

Barley typically contains between 10 and 11.5% nitrogen. A third of the proteins are kept as transport proteins in the endosperm's cell walls, which control mass transfer. A mere third of this protein makes it into the brewed beer. Despite the relatively small quantity of protein in beer, its quality can nonetheless be significantly impacted by it. Thus, proteins contribute significantly to the preservation of the head, but they can also play a significant role in the development of hazes in beer (Gupta et al., 2010). In any event, as the protein level of the barley rises, the amount of potential extract that can be obtained from malt falls by a similar amount (0.7 to 1.0%). Therefore, a maximum protein content of 11.5% in the dry matter is the standard commercial requirement.

4.11 AMINO ACIDS

Amino acids are the simplest building elements of nitrogen molecules (proteins). Although there are over 150 amino acids, only 20 are important for chemical compounds. This brief formula describes amino acids:

$$NH_2 - R - COOH$$

The amino group is formed by the -NH_2 group, while the acid is made up of the weakly dissociated COOH- (carbonyl) group. The "R" stands for the variably arranged main group. When water is discharged from the plant, amino acids are linked together to form lengthy unbranched chains. Only in the terminal amino acids does the -NH_2 group remain because throughout the process, the -NH group and the COOH group unite to create a HH-CO bond. There are more free terminal amino groups when the chains are shorter. However, as we will see, it is the free -NH_2 groups that are crucial for the yeast, and we must make sure that there is always enough free amino nitrogen (FAN) available for the yeast to eat. As a result, the following has several criteria for FAN: At least 200 mg FAN/L, or 20 mg FAN per 100/g, or 200 ppm, should be present in the cast wort. Yeast may metabolize amino acids to varying degrees of acceptability.

4.12 CONSTRUCTION OF PROTEINS

Living things build all proteins from unbranched chains of amino acids. The organism determines the order of the amino acids in the chain, and it is characteristic for that particular one. Molecular weights of over one million can be achieved by forming chains of up to 300 amino acids. The arrangement of amino acid molecules is divided into three categories:

- *Primary structure*, which is the overall molecule's sequenced arrangement of its amino acids.
- *Secondary structure*; the amino acid residues in proteins coil in the secondary structure, which is sometimes compared to a telephone cord, similarly to how the glucose residues coil in the amylose molecule.

- *Tertiary structure*, in which a sequence-defined ball is formed from a long, partially twisted protein molecule. Hydrogen bridges, electrostatic contacts, sulphur bridges, and other mechanisms are used to get the large molecules into a specified configuration while water is gathered for hydration. Proteins therefore transform into colloids, whose viscosity rises with molecule size.

Proteins respond in both an acidic and an alkaline manner because they are amphoteric; at this so-called isoelectric point (IP), they are neutral and have the lowest solubility. The handling of the nitrogenous compounds depends on the pH level during the brewing of beer. Large protein molecules become denatured and eventually coagulate when heated. As a result, the linkages deteriorate, a disorderly condition develops, and precipitation results. However, the size and structure of the molecule play a big role in this. In this category, which either does not dissolve at all in the wort or precipitates at the latest during wort boiling, the majority of barley protein (about 92%) may be found. According to Osborne, proteins are divided into several classes based on how soluble they are in aqueous solutions.

4.12.1 Glutelin

Approximately 30% of the protein in barley is glutelin, which only dissolves in weak alkali. This protein is nearly totally localized in the aleurone layer, is not subsequently broken down, and enters the wasted grains unchanged.

4.12.2 Prolamin

Hordein, a prolamin found in barley, makes up around 37% of the protein in the grain. It dissolves in 80% alcohol, and some of it ends up in the used grains.

4.12.3 Globulin

Edestin is the name of the barley globulin fraction. It dissolves in weak salt solution and also in the mash. It makes up around 15% of the protein in barley. Edestin is made up of four parts (a, 13, y, 6); however, the 13-globulin, which contains sulfur, does not entirely precipitate even after prolonged boiling and might cause haze in beer.

4.12.4 Albumin

Leucosin is the name given to barley albumin. It has a molecular weight of 70,000 on average and 16 distinct components. Since one Dalton (Da) equals the mass of one proton, the molecular mass and Dalton have the same value (mol. mass 70,000 = 70 kDa), which is how the molecular size is typically stated. Leucosin, which makes up about 11% of the protein in barley, dissolves in clean water. It totally precipitates after boiling.

Protein Z, which has a molecular weight of 40 kDa, and the lipid transfer protein, which has a molecular weight of 10 kDa, are both albumins and are recognized as the two key components of beer foam. Throughout the malting process, each of them goes through a number of alterations. In addition to these proteins, barley also contains glycoproteins, which result in the bonding of proteins with a carbohydrate, such as glucose, mannose, or galactose. These glycoproteins may be broken down during the malting process and enhance the beer's foam stabilizing effect (Kunze, 2004).

4.13 POLYPHENOLS

This is a broad word for substances that have an astringent, concentrated bitter taste and an action that causes protein to precipitate. They are distinguished chemically by molecules that include several phenol rings (polyphenols). Despite making up just 0.1 to 0.3% of the dry matter in barley, polyphenols can have a significant impact on the beer's flavor stability and shelf life due to their antioxidant properties.

Both the barley husk and the aleurone layer contain polyphenols. Therefore, emphasis is placed on barley with thin, finely wrinkled husks, or an attempt is made, in the event of thick-husked barley, to remove a sizable portion of this material in the maltings. Their concentration generally rises with the thickness of the husk. With regard to haze and anthocyanins and their early phases, we are particularly interested in flavan-3-ol in the case of polyphenols. Numerous varieties of fruit include anthocyanins, which are bitter artificial scents and colors that may change color based on the acidity of the fruit (pH value).

Antioxidants are a function of polyphenols. If they are oxidized, they lose their antioxidant function, and their harmful effects become more pronounced. Therefore, it's crucial to stop polyphenols from oxidizing in any way.

4.14 ENZYMES

In all living things, there are enzymes. A huge variety of enzymes are present in both yeast and barley. The various changes that take place during brewing and malting are entirely dependent on the activity of enzymes. Therefore, discussing enzymes, their structures, and their mechanisms is crucial at this point. High-molecular-weight proteins called enzymes operate as biocatalysts to either promote or significantly speed up specific processes. They control the course and speed of metabolic activities and are active even in extremely low concentrations.

The name of an enzyme is often formed by adding the suffix *-ase* to the end of the name of the substrate that is to be broken down. So, sucrase is the name of the enzyme that breaks down sugar (sucrose). Numerous enzymes are found in barley; however, most of them are only at trace levels. The majority of the enzymes in malt are created during the malting process.

4.15 HOPS

The hop is a perennial, dioecious climbing plant of the hemp family (*Humulus lupulus* L.), and a member of the Urticales order, which also contains the nettle family. The female plant's inflorescences are what are used in the brewery. These provide the beer with its bittering and fragrance components by way of bitter resins and ethereal oils. The dried hop cones of the female hop plant and any products manufactured from them that exclusively include hops-related ingredients are known as hops in the brewing industry. Hops are cultivated in specialized growing areas that provide the ideal circumstances for their growth. The hops are treated once they are harvested to preserve their value. When evaluating hops, the hop cone's composition and structure are crucial pieces of information (Palmer, 2001).

4.16 HOPS HARVESTING

The hops need to be dried and put into a shape that can be stored after harvest. Hop picking takes place at the end of August when the crop is technically mature and needs to be finished in 14 days. The female inflorescences, or cones, are harvested by removing the hop bine's fasteners from the support wires. Today, hop-picking machines are used exclusively in the harvest of hops.

Water makes up around 75 to 80% of the harvested hop. The hops must be dried right away since they cannot be kept in this state. On belt dryers or in small businesses, drying is done in batches in kilns. The hops are meticulously dried to a water content of 8 to 12% at a temperature of no more than 50°C. The hops are then compressed, or pushed, into larger or looser bales (pockets). The hops cannot be kept for an extended period of time, even in this state, without losing quality (Moir, 2000).

The bittering value quickly declines as a result of oxygen action, moisture impact, and heating, and other negative effects also take place. Therefore, it is necessary to stabilize the hops right away.

Only a tiny portion of the harvested hops are added as natural hops; the majority are converted into extract and pellets. In every scenario, there is a period of time between harvesting and processing during which the hops must be kept from further deterioration. To do this, dried hops are formed into ballots that are around 1.1 meters long and 0.6 meters in diameter using hydraulic presses, which are then placed inside sacks and stitched shut. The finished ballot is roughly 65 kilograms in weight. Compression reduces the amount of air that can reach the hops, which makes it harder for them to absorb moisture. The storage of the ballots has long since been altered to an easily stackable, right-angled form (60 × 60 × 120 cm), which has taken the place of the loose bales, in order to make the most use of the storage capacity. The right-angled bales have served as the foundation for cold storage, which is efficient and keeps the hops' value and quality high (Kunze, 2004).

4.17 HOP CONE STRUCTURE

Although there are separate male and female plants in the hop plant, only the female plants are grown by hop producers. These plants begin to produce inflorescences in their second year, and because of their form, these inflorescences are known as hop cones.

The stem or strig should be small. Egg-shaped bracts with yellowish-green leaves that are more yellow at the base than the tip can be found. A cone-shaped arrangement of bracts is present. On the bracteoles, which are found between the sprig and the bracts, are lupulin glands, which are visible as a yellow, clingy powder. It occurs

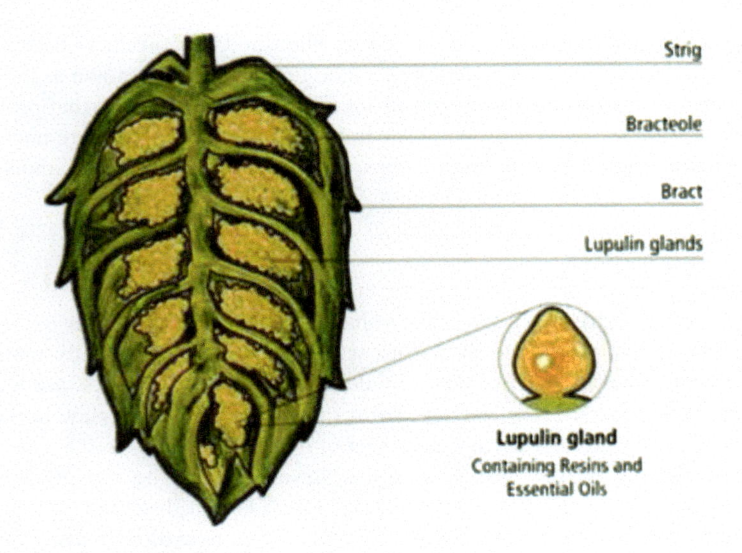

FIGURE 4.2 Hop Cone Structure

in beaker-shaped glands where ethereal oils and resins are secreted. A membrane covers the gland to stop the contents from leaking out. The gland gets broken off when it is disturbed. Except for the polyphenols, all the components of hops that are useful for brewing beer are found in the lupulin glands.

4.18 COMPOSITION

The hops' chemical makeup has a huge impact on the quality of the beer that is made with them. The hop dry weight is made up of:

Bitter substances	18.5%
Hop oil	0.5%
Polyphenols	3.5%
Protein	20.0%
Minerals	8.0%

Cellulose and other substances unrelated to the manufacturing of beer make up the remaining portion. The bitter compounds and hop oil are the most crucial ingredients in the creation of beer.

The growing lupulin gland of the hop plant already secretes a β-acid that is only somewhat bitter at this early stage of development. A portion of these β-acids is transformed into the much more bitter α-acids throughout the maturing phase. The weather has a big impact on this conversion, which only applies to some of the β-acids. For instance, hot and dry maturation seasons hinder this conversion process more than cold, wet summers do.

The most crucial bonds for the bittering of the beer are α-acids or humulones. These bonds, nevertheless, are uniformly flat. The cohumulone, one of the bonds, plays a more detrimental effect in beer bittering. Hop producers currently try to develop mostly varieties with a low proportion of cohumulone since the quantity of the α-acids generated and their composition are varietal characteristics. Less than 20 to 25% of cohumulone in the α-acid content is the target percentage. In the case of aroma hops, the α-acid level ranges from 4 to 5% on average.

Some hop cultivars, such Northern Brewer, have greater α-acid content (6 to 9%); however, they also usually contain larger proportions of cohumulone (over 30% of the α-acids). They are thus more bitter, but since they contain more cohumulone, they are often not as high quality as other types with a smaller concentration of cohumulone.

There are some new hop cultivars being grown that have an α-acid concentration between 15 and 16%. Nugget, Target, Hallertauer Magnum, and Hallertauer Taurus are a few examples of these high α-types, and the proportion of high-alpha varieties is steadily rising (Bober et al., 2020).

The originally insoluble α-acids are eventually converted into soluble iso α-acids during wort boiling (isomerization), which, aside from precipitating during cooling

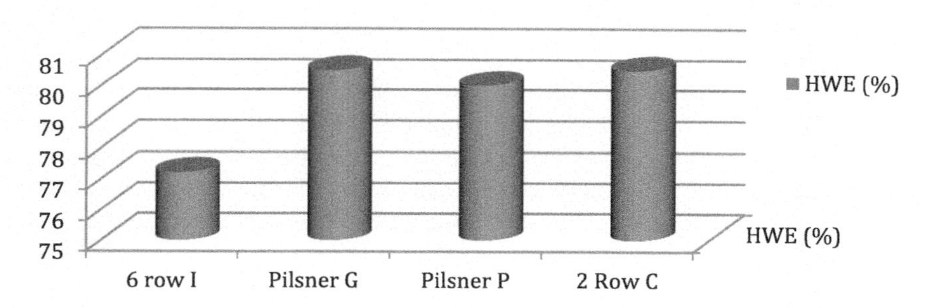

FIGURE 4.3 Hot Water Extract (HWE%) of Different Malts

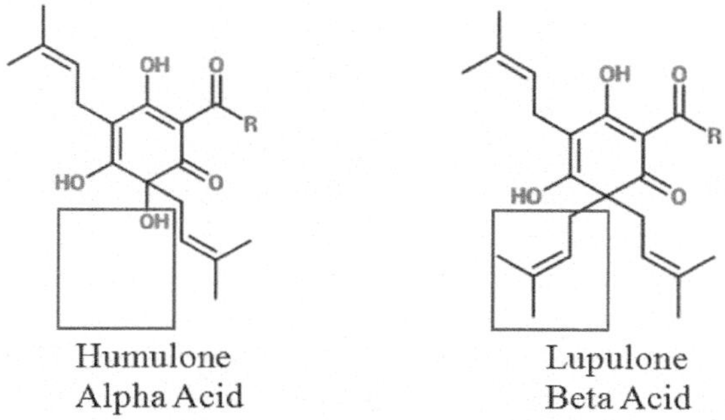

OH O R HO O OH

Humulone
Alpha Acid

OH O R HO O

Lupulone
Beta Acid

FIGURE 4.4 Structure of Alpha and Beta Acids of Hops

and fermentation, enters the final beer and contributes to the bitterness. Strongly hopped beers should have higher head retention since the bitter ingredients are extremely surface active, which increases the beer's foam stability. The bitter ingredients help prevent the growth of microorganisms in beer; nevertheless, this bacteriostatic effect is not very strong and does not take the place of the necessary steps required to establish beer stability.

However, the membrane covering the lupulin gland is permeable and only offers minimal protection for the contents, and the α-acids do not last. The α-acids are gradually broken down by the effects of oxygen, higher temperatures, and increased humidity. Therefore, it can be projected that at a storage temperature of 18°C, up to 25% of the α-acids will have been broken down in two months. This indicates that the breakdown process starts right after the formation of α-acids and their maturity.

As a result, it becomes necessary to keep the hops cool, dry, and air-free until they are processed. The α- and β-acids are only converted to the hard resins, which no longer have any use for brewing. Old hops have a cheesy fragrance because valeric acid's side chain breaks off when the bitter chemicals do.

The most important and distinctive part of a hop plant is its resins. Due to their antibacterial qualities, they strengthen the biological stability of the beer, give it its bitter flavor, and enhance foam stability. Individual hop resins have highly varying bittering qualities, as was already noted. The β-acid fraction is outweighed by the α-acid's contribution to bitterness by a factor of nine.

The α-acid is by far the most crucial element, and it also largely defines the hop's trading value. As a result, producing and cultivating high-alpha cultivars has received a lot of attention in recent years. High-alpha hop cultivars with α-acid content of 12 to 16% and cohumulone content of less than 25% have just entered the market. A market share of 8.8% is held by the production of high-alpha, high-bittering hop cultivars worldwide. About one-third of a beer's bitterness comes from the (non-specific) soft resins, which are another group of bitter flavors (Bober et al., 2020).

4.19 HOP OIL

Hops have a hop oil content of 0.5 to 1.2%, which denotes 200 to 250 distinct ethereal substances that become more volatile when heated. The lupulin gland secretes them from the developing plant, giving the hops their distinctive flavor. Hop oil falls within the categories of hydrocarbons and bonds containing oxygen.

Only with the use of gas chromatographic analyses can the proportions of the various components of hop oil be recorded. The bonds here appear as chit. However, no inferences can be made from this information about how the various scent components combine to produce the final aroma. As a result, determining the hops' quality is still primarily done by hand.

Hop oil has a range of compositions that depend on the variety. It is possible to distinguish between fragrance elements that tend to be more fruity and those that are more floral. Hop oil has a variety of little-known chemicals with obscure names that we won't address here, but three in particular are myrcene, linalool, and nonanal (Schonberger & Kostelecky, 2011).

Myrcene is an unfavorable low-boiling monoterpene that gives the hop fragrance a particular sharpness and gives the beer a rough and disagreeable flavor. Linalool, which has lately grown significantly in importance, acts quite differently. The $R^{(-)}$ linalool and the $S^{(+)}$ linalool are two isomeric molecules present in this hop oil. About 90% of the linalool in hops exists as R(+) linalool; however, the ratio shifts throughout the brewing process in favor of $S^{(+)}$ linalool (52:48).

The very flavor- and aroma-active compound $R^{(-)}$ linalool has been consistently demonstrated to be the source of the distinctively floral orange blossom and geranium aromas. Valuable scent components are lost during the brewing process as a result of the partial transfer of the floral $R^{(-)}$ linalool to the less distinctive $S^{(+)}$ linalool. Whirlpool hopping is considered the most successful hopping technique, although it results in a loss of bitterness.

It is also possible to create pure hop aroma compounds, such as $R^{(-)}$ linalool, and add them to the beer using specific fractioning techniques (= PHAS, Barth & Sohn, Nuremberg). However, this does not adhere to the Purity Law.

Examples of fragrance components include the sesquiterpenes β-caryophyllene, β-farnesene, and humulene or its epoxide. The hop oil evaporates more and more as it boils in the brewing house. Afterwards, a portion of the hop is added to beers in which an aromatic hop flavor and fragrance are valued, relinquishing a portion of the isomerized α-acid in order to retain at least some of the fragrant hop oil. α-acid levels of just 4 to 6%, a targeted proportion of cohumulone of less than 20%, and the greatest possible proportions of humulene and farnesene in the hop oil are the characteristics of so-called aroma hops, which are kinds with a fine scent (Schonberger & Kostelecky, 2011).

In Germany, the percentage of aroma hops has climbed from 48% to 63% of the overall crop during the past ten years. Hallertauer Mittelfrueh, Hallertauer Tradition, Hersbrucker Spaet, Opal, Perle, Saphir, Smaragd, Spalter, Spatter Select, and Tettnanger are some types of German aroma hops.

4.20 POLYPHENOLS IN HOPS

Hops have a dry matter content of 2 to 5% polyphenol, which is nearly completely found in the sprig and bracts. For the brewer, polyphenols have the following crucial qualities: They have an anti-oxidizing action, an astringent taste, and the ability to mix and precipitate with complex proteins. They also have the ability to oxidize to reddish-brown compounds called phlobaphenes and interact with iron salts to generate black compounds.

Due to these characteristics, the polyphenols have a role in the haze production and the flavor and color of beer. The term "polyphenols" refers to a class of chemicals that can range in complexity from simple to complex and includes several phenyl groups.

They are made up of a combination of catechins, flavonols, tannins, and anthocyanogens. The anthocyanogens (proanthocyanidins) are the most significant of these polyphenols, in terms of both quantity and quality. Anthocyanogens make up around 80% of the polyphenol in hops. The anthocyanogens found in malt, which are mostly found in the aleurone layer, are structurally quite similar to those found in hops.

Eighty percent of the anthocyanogens in a typical mash come from the malt, and 20% from the hops (Karabin et al., 2016).

Hop's polyphenols differ from malt's primarily due to their higher degree of condensation and higher level of reactivity. The anti-oxidizing properties of polyphenols make them beneficial for flavor stability. It is crucial to avoid any kind of oxidation since the anti-oxidizing action vanishes with oxidation.

Xanthohumol and isoxanthohumol are two more polyphenols found in hops. These chemicals are said to have anti-oxidative and anti-carcinogenic characteristics. A method (Xan) has been devised to attain a xanthohumol concentration of 1–3 mg p/I in the final beer since only very minute levels of xanthohumol, far under 0.2 mg p/I, have been found in finished beer made using traditional procedures (Magalhaes et al., 2009).

4.21 NITROGEN SUBSTANCES

Nitrogen makes up about 12 to 20% of the dry weight of hops, and 30 to 50% of this nitrogen enters the beer. Hop protein is not necessary for beer production (foam generation, palate fullness) due to its low concentration. In the process of making beer, the other elements of hops—carbohydrates, organic acids, and inorganic substances—are irrelevant.

4.22 HOP VARIETIES

With a high market price, hops are by far the most expensive raw ingredient used in the making of beer. As a result, choosing the right types for growing and dealing with hops is crucial. The fact that aroma hops with a low bittering value are also in great demand, in addition to hops with a high bittering value, has also been brought up.

The pleasant hop aroma, a cohumulone percentage of less than 20%, and a high proportion of finely fragrant components set apart aroma varieties (caryophyllia, farnesene). Although they only contain 2.5 to 5% α-acid, they are occasionally traded at greater prices. For example, Perle, Spatter Select, and Hallertauer Tradition are desirable aromatic hops. Bittering cultivars are identified by their high α-acid content, which can range from above 10% to up to 15%. Cohumulone should make up no more than 25% of the composition of a good high-alpha cultivar.

Hops are initially recognized by the growing location and then by the variety: for example, Hallertauer: Hallertauer Tradition or Elbe-Saale Hallertauer Tradition, as the quality of the hop is influenced by both the variety and the growing region (Schonberger & Kostelecky, 2011).

The α-acid concentration also depends on the harvesting year and might exhibit dramatic changes depending on the weather in any given year.

Hallertauer Merkur (10–14% α-acid, 17–22% cohumulone) and Hallertauer Herkules are two new high-alpha types (12–17% α-acid, 32–38% cohumulone). Hallertauer Opal (5–8% α-acid), Hallertauer Saphir (2–4.5% α-acid), and Hallertauer Smaragd (4–6% α -acid) are new aroma hop varieties (cohumulone content for all 3 varieties: 12–18%). Most people consider the bitterness of hop cultivars with a low cohumulone level to be milder and more agreeable. Low-cohumulone-content hops provide improved head retention.

4.23 HOP PRODUCTS

Because of the enormous benefits that the introduction of hop products offers, the number of breweries that employ hop cones is steadily declining. It is feasible to maintain a consistent bitterness in the beer by using hop products.

Products made from hops may be kept for virtually always. Therefore, in good harvest years, it is feasible to buy the reserve hops. One is also no longer reliant on the vast price differences on the hop market.

Utilizing hop products might increase the output of bitterness. Lower transportation and storage expenses result from using hop products. A hop separator is not required when using hop products. Products containing hops can be dosed automatically (O'Rourke, 2003).

4.24 HOP PELLETS

Pelletization is an extremely efficient method of maintaining the contents of hops. The dried hops are ground into a powder in this procedure, which is followed by compression into pellets. Hops are easily introduced when they are in pellet form since they are free flowing.

Three different hop-pellet types exist.

4.25 PELLET TYPE 90

In order to create type-90 pellets, 100 kilogrammes of intact hop cones are converted into 90 kg of powder, which contains all the essential components of the original hops. The type-90 hop pellets are produced by first thoroughly drying the hop cones with air at 20 to 25°C, followed by hot air at 40 to 50°C, to a water content of 7 to 9% and then milling to a powder with a grain size of 1 to 5mm. In a pelleting device with a molding die that includes cylindrical holes, this powder is combined and formed into pellets. The ground-up material is compressed to create the usual cylindrical pellet shape.

The hops warm up throughout this procedure, which may cause a decline in their price. Therefore, it's crucial to keep the temperature below 50°C. The pellets are chilled in the subsequent process, kept in silos, and packaged without the presence of air; the package is then filled with CO_2 or nitrogen as a protective gas. To keep the content's quality high, this is essential. The pellets should be stored at a low temperature of 1–3°C; at higher temperatures, the bitterness decreases, and hard resin forms, causing a value decline (O'Rourke, 2003).

4.26 ENRICHED PELLETS (TYPE 45)

The fact that the lupulin glands contain all the resin and oil allows for the production of lupulin-enriched pellets (type 45). These naturally occur in particles that are around 0.15 mm. It is necessary to divide a portion of the bract and strig fraction.

Machines for milling and sieving are utilized for this. However, a lupulin gland has to be hard and lose its adhesive force in order to be physically processed, so the liquid inside needs to solidify. Therefore, milling and sieving are carried out at extremely low temperatures, preferably around –35°C (Kunze, 2004).

4.27 HOP EXTRACTS

Extraction is the process of removing certain components from a solid using a suitable solvent. However, in the food sector, interest typically extends beyond the simple dissolving procedure, and the solution is subsequently concentrated to the necessary level by solvent evaporation. In other words, the solvent just serves as a vehicle for the compounds to be separated from the solid.

Nowadays, liquid CO_2 and ethanol are used as the solvents for making hop extracts because the long-established method of extraction using methylene chloride has been discontinued for environmental preservation. Because the hop resins and oils are entirely dissolved by the two solvents now in use, they are both especially well suited for the extraction of hops (O'Rourke, 2003).

4.28 YEAST

Yeast is a unicellular microorganism that can produce the energy it requires through fermentation, both when there is oxygen present (aerobic) and when there isn't (anaerobic). During the brewing of beer, yeast ferments the sugar in the wort to produce alcohol and carbon dioxide. This is accomplished by using yeast fungus of the species *Saccharomyces cerevisiae* for top-fermenting beers and *Saccharomyces carlsbergensis* for bottom-fermenting beers in the brewery. Pure-culture brewers' yeasts are produced by methodically isolating and growing a few of these yeasts. Other *Saccharomyces cerevisiae* strains are employed as distiller or bakers' yeasts. The yeast *Saccharomyces ellipsoideus* is used to make wine (Palmer, 2001).

Understanding the structures and composition of yeasts, their metabolism, and their development is crucial since they not only create alcohol but also have a significant impact on the flavor and character of beer. Different kinds and races of culture yeasts are present with a variety of distinguishing characteristics.

4.29 YEAST METABOLISM

The yeast cell, like all other cells, needs energy and food to carry out its vital metabolic functions and to manufacture new cell components. Like all other living things, yeast uses respiration to obtain the energy needed to complete these tasks. The quantity of energy obtained by respiration is particularly high since glucose is completely converted to CO_2 and H_2O, the lowest-energy compounds, and more energy cannot be obtained through breakdown.

The food that is ingested, such as sugar, is completely broken down into CO_2 and water during respiration:

$$C_6H_{12}O_6 + 6O_2 \rightarrow 6H_2O + 6CO_2$$

Yeast is the only living creature that changes to an alcoholic fermentation in the presence of sugar; in this process (to summarize), glucose is transformed to alcohol (ethanol) and CO_2.

$$C_6H_{12}O_6 \rightarrow C_2H_5OH + 2CO_2$$

Numerous reactions take place one after the other to break down glucose into alcohol or, in the case of respiration, CO_2 and water. A specific enzyme catalyses each stage of the process. These enzymes are incorporated into certain cell structures inside the yeast cell. As a result, the cytoplasm contains the enzymes for glycolysis and alcoholic fermentation, whereas the mitochondria have the enzymes for respiration.

The cell wall's integrated proteins transfer the organic materials required for respiration and fermentation across the membrane. Only compounds for which proper transport pathways are present can be taken up by the yeast cell. Once more, this is based on the yeast's range of enzymes (Ferreira et al., 2010).

The metabolism of carbohydrates, nitrogen, lipids, and inorganic substances in the yeast cell is intricate. Only a very tiny portion of the sugar present in the wort will be kept as a reserve in the form of glycogen and trehalose, which means that the primary purpose of the carbohydrate metabolism is to supply energy through respiration and fermentation.

The primary function of the nitrogen metabolism, like that of fat and inorganic material metabolisms, is to replenish the components of the cell, in which both the creation and breakdown processes play a significant role. The yeast also produces and stores glycerine. Glycerine is an osmotically active intercellular molecule that keeps the enzymes working even when there is little water activity. As the initial wort content rises, more glycerine is produced (Palmer, 2001).

Yeasts typically bud to reproduce. They are also known as budding anger because of this. A daughter cell's nucleus, created by division, travels through a tiny bubble-like protuberance from the mother cell during budding, and a complete daughter cell is created. Some yeast strains entirely separate the mother and daughter cells, as a result of which the mother cell's bud scars are visible. Up to 20 scars can be found on old yeast cells. Top-fermenting strains still remain connected and the form bud colonies.

There are four different stages of yeast growth: lag, log, stationary, and decline.

4.30 BREWING YEAST

The yeast strains that are most frequently utilized in breweries come in a variety of distinct strains. Top-fermenting yeasts (*Saccharomyces cerevisiae*) and bottom-fermenting yeasts (*Saccharomyces carlsbergensis*) are the two main categories in brewing practice.

Under a microscope, top- and bottom-fermenting yeasts can be distinguished based on how they behave throughout the budding process. Top-fermenting yeasts generate chains of budded cells, whereas bottom-fermenting yeasts almost exclusively exist as single cells or pairs of cells.

The mother and daughter cells of top-fermenting yeasts stay connected to one another for a longer period of time, and, as a result, branching chains of cells are created. When the division is finished, the mother and daughter cells in bottom-fermenting yeasts separate. Both top- and bottom-fermenting yeasts have the same cell structure (White & Zainasheff, 2010).

The fermentation of trisaccharide raffinose is the primary physiological difference between top- and bottom-fermenting yeast. Due to their wide range of enzymes, bottom-fermenting yeasts can utilize raffinose completely, but top-fermenting yeasts can only ferment a third of the trisaccharide.

Other changes can be seen in respiratory and fermentative metabolism and spore-forming capacity. While top-fermenting yeasts exhibit a prominent respiratory metabolism, bottom-fermenting yeasts have a significantly higher fermentative metabolism. In line with this, top-fermenting yeast strains produce a lot more yeast after fermentation than bottom-fermenting strains do. Compared to top-fermenting strains, bottom-fermenting yeasts have a lower enzyme content. Bottom-fermenting yeasts also have a restricted capacity to produce ascospore. They produce spores more slowly and less often than top-fermenting strains. Spore production is completely absent when fermentation is carried out normally.

Brewing yeast strains are given the designations "top fermenting" and "bottom fermenting" based on how they emerge during fermentation. During fermentation, top-fermenting yeasts climb to the top, whereas bottom-fermenting yeasts sink to the bottom as fermentation progresses. At the conclusion of fermentation, top-fermenting yeasts also sink to the bottom, but considerably later than bottom-fermenting strains. As long as open containers are being utilized, they are collected there at the end of the primary fermentation (Palmer, 2001).

The various flocculation behaviors exhibited by bottom-fermenting yeasts are another crucial trait. Thus, powdery and flocculent yeasts are two categories for bottom-fermenting yeasts. When it comes to powdery yeasts, the cells stay very finely split in the medium during fermentation and only begin to gently sink to the bottom when fermentation is complete. The flocculent yeast's cells quickly group together to create sizable flocs before settling quickly. A yeast's ability to flocculate is genetically determined. Yeasts that ferment at the top do not create flocs.

The capacity of a yeast to flocculate is extremely useful. While powdered yeasts and top-fermenting yeasts generate a turbid beer with a higher level of attenuation, flocculent yeasts produce a clear beer that is less fully fermented.

Regarding fermentation temperature, top- and bottom-fermenting yeasts are different. Between 4 and 12°C is the temperature for bottom-fermenting yeast fermentations. The temperature range for top-fermenting yeasts is 14 to 25°C. The brewer is in charge of controlling the temperature (Pires & Branyik, 2015).

4.31 WATER

The primary raw material used in the manufacturing of beer in terms of quantity is water. Only a portion of the necessary water is utilized to make beer, with the remainder going toward washing, rinsing, and other uses. Because the quality of the water has an impact on the quality of the beer produced, the supply and preparation of the water are particularly crucial to the brewer.

The requirements for the quality of drinking water are also continuously increasing. Water must meet at least the same quality standards as drinking water in order to be used in the manufacturing of beer. The brewing of beer exerts additional demands on the quality of the water. Businesses have been obliged to reduce their water use due to rising expenses for obtaining fresh water and disposing of waste water. Between 5 and 8 hl/hr of fresh water, on average, are used in breweries. Small breweries often consume more water than large ones.

4.32 BREWING WATER

Salts are always there, dissolved in water. They are no longer present as salts and are instead virtually entirely present as dissociated ions due to their significant dilution. Therefore, referring to dissolved ions is more appropriate.

During mashing, when these ions have their initial contact with the malt components, the majority do not react. On the other hand, certain ions interact with specific malt constituents. As a consequence, ions that are chemically reactive may be distinguished from those that lack chemical activity (Dehrmann & Cameron, 2011).

All ions that do not undergo chemical interactions with malt constituents and instead flow into beer unmodified are referred to as chemically inactive ions. They can have either a positive or a negative impact on beer flavor when present in big numbers. As a result, sodium chloride (NaCl), for instance, imparts a more nuanced flavor. The salts sodium chloride, potassium chloride (KCl), sodium sulfate (Na_2SO_4), and potassium sulfate (K_2SO_4), among others, are chemically inactive. However, some of these inert ions have an impact on certain brewing processes. The ions listed here are chemically inactive, but only inasmuch as they don't react with the parts of the malt that they come into contact with when making wort. During the mashing process, a variety of ions (chemically reactive) in the brewing water interact with the components of the malt, changing the acidity (pH value) of the beer (Palmer, 2001).

TABLE 4.1
Physicochemical Properties of Beers

Parameter	LB	CLB	WB	CWB	AB	DB	BBB	KB
pH	5.62	5.73	5.52	5.59	5.12	5.07	5.21	5.13
Original Extract (°Plato)	12.5	12.3	12.3	12.1	12.5	11.9	12.5	12.5
Final Gravity (°Plato)	2.6	2.4	3.0	2.9	3.2	2.9	2.6	2.6
Attenuation	79.2	79.8	75.6	76	74.4	75.6	79.2	79.2
Alcohol Content	5.4	5.4	5.1	5.06	5.1	4.95	5.4	5.4
Bitterness	18	18	17	18	17	16	17	17

4.33 pH VALUE

The pH has a significant impact on a number of beer manufacturing processes. Enzymes, for instance, have an ideal pH value and are less active at lower pH levels. Enzymes govern the majority of the processes involved in the creation of malt and beer.

The dissociated salts and organic molecules included in beer products determine the pH level. These came from the water, malt, additives, and hops. The chemically reactive ions present in the water encounter soluble malt components and form new compounds. The majority of brewing operations move forward more quickly and more efficiently the more acidic the pH (Dehrmann & Cameron, 2011).

Therefore, throughout the production process, the pH should be as low as possible. Difficulties are to be expected at higher pH levels. The salts that are chemically reactive are separated into pH-increasing and pH-decreasing ions. It is preferable to speak of pH-raising and pH-lowering ions or of acidifying (pH-lowering ions) and acidity neutralizing (pH-raising ions) since the salts in brewing water mostly reside in the dissociated state as ions.

4.34 WATER IMPROVEMENTS

Water quality needs to be checked on a regular basis, and it's crucial to consider what needs to be altered or improved. The method of treatment is determined by the intended use of the water. So, for instance, it doesn't matter if the water includes bacteria if it will be utilized as boiler feed water; what matters is the quantity and kind of dissolved salts. It works exactly the other way around for cleansing water. Therefore, it is important to distinguish between the processes used to remove dissolved chemicals, microorganisms, and dissolved gases, as well as suspended particles and reduced residual alkalinity in brewing water.

4.35 REFERENCES

Bamforth, C. (Ed.). (2006). *Brewing: New technologies*. Woodhead Publishing.

Bober, A., Liashenko, M., Protsenko, L., Slobodyanyuk, N., Matseiko, L., Yashchuk, N., & Mushtruk, M. (2020). Biochemical composition of the hops and quality of the finished beer. *Potravinarstvo*, *14*(1).

Dehrmann, F. M., & Cameron, A. (2011). *The importance of water and water quality in brewing*. SAAFost (SAB).

Ferreira, I. M. P. L. V. O., Pinho, O., Vieira, E., & Tavarela, J. G. (2010). Brewer's Saccharomyces yeast biomass: Characteristics and potential applications. *Trends in Food Science & Technology*, *21*(2), 77–84.

Gupta, M., Abu-Ghannam, N., & Gallaghar, E. (2010). Barley for brewing: Characteristic changes during malting, brewing and applications of its by-products. *Comprehensive Reviews in Food Science and Food Safety*, *9*(3), 318–328.

Karabin, M., Hudcova, T., Jelínek, L., & Dostalek, P. (2016). Biologically active compounds from hops and prospects for their use. *Comprehensive Reviews in Food Science and Food Safety*, *15*(3), 542–567.

Kok, Y. J., Ye, L., Muller, J., Ow, D. S. W., & Bi, X. (2019). Brewing with malted barley or raw barley: What makes the difference in the processes? *Applied Microbiology and Biotechnology*, *103*(3), 1059–1067.

Kunze, W. (2004). *Brewing malting* (pp. 18–152). VLB.
Magalhaes, P. J., Carvalho, D. O., Cruz, J. M., Guido, L. F., & Barros, A. A. (2009). Fundamentals and health benefits of xanthohumol, a natural product derived from hops and beer. *Natural Product Communications*, *4*(5), 1934578X0900400501.
Moir, M. (2000). Hops-a millennium review. *Journal of the American Society of Brewing Chemists*, *58*(4), 131–146.
O'Rourke, T. (2003). Hops and hop products. *Brew International*, *3*(1), 21–25.
Palmer, J. J. (2001). *How to brew: Ingredients, methods, recipes, and equipment for brewing beer at home*. Defenestrative Publishing Company.
Pires, E., & Branyik, T. (2015). *Biochemistry of beer fermentation* (pp. 4–7). Springer International Publishing.
Schonberger, C., & Kostelecky, T. (2011). 125th anniversary review: The role of hops in brewing. *Journal of the Institute of Brewing*, *117*(3), 259–267.
Schwarz, P., & Li, Y. (2011). Malting and brewing uses of barley. In *Barley: Production, improvement, and uses* (pp. 478–521). Blackwell.
White, C., & Zainasheff, J. (2010). *Yeast: The practical guide to beer fermentation*. Brewers Publications.

5 Additives Used in Brewing and Fermentation for Beer Production

Competition in the beer market is increasing day by day, so breweries are under pressure to lower the cost of beer production and also to diversify their offerings by creating new products with different ingredients in response to consumer demand. These new products are produced by using different substitutes (adjuncts) to brewing raw materials and also by using various additives. Up to 85 to 90% of beer produced today across the globe is thought to have adjuncts. The use of adjuncts can have both positive and negative effects on the quality of the finished product. Therefore, it is essential to understand the effects of particular adjuncts on the various characteristics of beer in order to ensure appropriate use. With the proper selection of an adjunct, the shelf life of beer can be increased, and the colors can be made lighter. By modifying the sugar and amino acid spectra in wort, the flavor profile can also be modified.

The use of adjuncts varies greatly across different continents, though. Between 10 and 30% of malt is replaced by unmalted grains in European nations, 40 to 50% or more in U.S. and Australian countries, and between 50 and 75% in Africa (Annemuller & Manger, 2013).

The use of unmalted grains also decreases the need to process barley, which may be impacted by unfavorable weather conditions in specific years and can even lessen malt shortages on the global market (Goode et al., 2005). Native grains are typically utilized as a supplement to local agriculture. In Africa, sorghum is the most popular auxiliary crop, followed by corn and rice in Asia. The two adjuncts that are most often utilized in Europe are barley and maize (Annemuller & Manger, 2013).

Beer is a product that pairs well with various tastes: herbal extracts for medicinal or aromatic purposes, honey, sugar, coffee, and other ingredients. Additionally, it goes well with sweet fruits like raspberries, wild plums, and cherries. The practice of blending various supplements with beer extends back to the earliest times, when the goal was to create a drink that would stand out and be distinctive while also covering up flaws brought on by subpar manufacturing circumstances. *Artemisia vulgaris*, *Juniperus communis*, *Melissa officinalis*, *Mentha spicata*, *Origanum vulgare*, *Pimpinella anisum*, *Rosmarinus officinalis*, *Thymus serpyllum*, and other herbs have all been added to the brew. *Acorus calamus*, *Cinnamomum verum*, and *Hypericum perforatum* are plants that have been used to enhance the beneficial properties of beer.

DOI: 10.1201/b22906-5

With the inclusion of extractive plant isolates, there are now many new, unique sorts of beer. German wheat beer is enhanced with lemon juice, raspberry syrup, and specific herbal extracts, whereas comparable Belgian beers are enhanced with orange juice and coriander extract. Mestreechs Aajt from Denmark is a sweet beer with a little mustard flavor. The ginger-flavored beer known as ginger beer is made in Denmark, England, and the United States. The manufacture of particular kinds of beer is likewise not behind in France. Pietra Brewery creates a peculiar sweet beer with the flavor of chestnuts, while brewery Nesle in Normandy makes beer Epinoir with the addition of buckwheat. A unique brand of coconut beer is made in India, and Mexican *negra* beer gets its sweet flavor from a combination of plants and bitter chocolate. On the basis of the German Carlsberg Brewery, one may determine the true scope of this occurrence. Carlsberg has apparently introduced Karla, a beer with the addition of fruit juice, vitamins, folic acid, and lecithin, in an effort to appeal to the female portion of the population. It can be used as a prophylactic against many ailments because it is a natural substance that improves overall health.

The use of adjuncts, though, can have unfavorable effects as well. These risks can be reduced during the production of wort and beer by using appropriate processing techniques and commercially available enzymatic preparations.

5.1 MALT SUBSTITUTES

The preferred cereal grain used in conventional brewing techniques is malted barley. Malt has enough enzyme capacity to catabolize more starch. As a result, for financial reasons, certain regions of the world substitute unmalted grain for a portion of the malt, often between 15 and 20%. The term "raw grain" refers to this unmalted cereal, which is more affordable than the comparatively expensive malt. Preference is given to the grain varieties that are grown in greater quantities in the region, particularly maize, rice, and sorghum, which is particularly popular in Africa. It is reasonable to assume that between 85 and 90% of all beer made globally contains raw grain or an adjunct. Adjuncts are forbidden in beers made in accordance with the German *Reinheitsgebot*.

During the malting process, barley is altered to guarantee that biochemical alterations take place inside the grain that produce crucial enzymes, sugars, and proteins needed to produce wort. The base grist material for the majority of beers is malted barley, although the brewing industry is well versed in the partial substitution of barley with grain adjuncts, including wheat, maize, and rice.

Brewing with partially unmalted grains has grown to be a popular choice for cutting costs and carbon emissions because malting is an energy-intensive operation. Nearly half the carbon footprint associated with malt production 217 kg CO_2eq/t is attributable to the malting process, while the remaining 241 kg CO_2 eq/t are attributable to the farming of malting barley. The carbon footprint of the malting and brewing process may be significantly reduced by using unmalted adjuncts (Yorke et al., 2021).

Production of barley is expected to be significantly impacted by global climate change. Extreme weather events may result in significant drops in barley yields globally, with a possible loss of 17% under the worst circumstances, according to crop and economic models. According to some forecasts (Xie et al., 2018), the price of beer might rise by 193% by 2099 as a result of a decline in the world's supply of barley.

Therefore, using a variety of other ingredients may help ensure the supply of raw materials for brewing during a period of anticipated climate change. For instance, it has been anticipated that the US and China's maize yields will not be significantly negatively impacted by climate change (Li et al., 2011).

Over time, the definition of an adjunct has evolved. Currently, sources of extract other than malt are referred to as adjuncts. Depending on their state of matter, adjuncts can be classified as either solids or liquids. Barley, corn, rice, and (less importantly) wheat, oats, sorghum, rye, and triticale are included in the first category, together with unmalted pseudocereals (buckwheat, amaranth, and quinoa), cassava, teff, and granulated sugar (sucrose). All must be hydrolyzed during the mashing process using malt or exogenous microbial enzymes, with the exception of granulated sugar. They are referred to as mash vessel adjuncts for this reason. Hydrolyzed starch syrups (wort extenders), sucrose-based syrups made from sugar cane or sugar beet, malt extracts, and syrups made from hydrolyzed cereals are all examples of liquid adjuncts (wort replacements). The composition of the latter is comparable to that of brewing wort and includes minerals in addition to carbs (Habschied et al., 2020).

Unmalted adjuncts are frequently used in the brewing industry because they are a different, more affordable source of extract and because of the unique functionality they add to the brewing process and final beers. By minimizing the need for the malting process and its associated expenditures, costs can be reduced. Additionally, switching up potentially pricey barley malt for less expensive regionally acquired grains might result in cost savings. Thus, local factors affecting the availability and pricing of raw materials have a significant impact on the choice of unmalted grains across the worldwide sector. In Europe and the United States, barley and corn are the most often utilized auxiliary grains, whereas rice is more widely employed in Asia. Some of the top worldwide beer companies' quality characteristics are dependent on the adjuncts they employ in their formulas. Brewers use adjuncts to alter beer quality (such as flavor, froth, and colloidal stability) as well as to create new, unique beverages with a variety of desirable attributes (Kok et al., 2019).

It can be difficult to brew with unmalted cereal adjuncts, especially at higher concentrations, and a deeper knowledge of the reasons limiting the upward absorption rates of unmalted adjunct materials is needed. The functionality and processability of the grain must be guaranteed when adding large concentrations of adjunct material, and there should be no detrimental effects on output or product quality.

The reduction in amylolytic, cytolytic, and proteolytic enzymatic activity in the grist (since these enzyme systems are activated and synthesized during the malting process) is the biggest drawback in terms of processability when incorporating unmalted adjuncts. The activities of these three enzyme systems during malting and mashing affect the wort's chemical makeup and the effectiveness of extract recovery in brewing. The performance of the brewing process and the quality of the produced beer will be impacted by the variable biochemical makeup of grain ingredients. The flavor profile of adjunct beers may be impacted by differences in the content of unmalted adjuncts and a lack of adequate enzyme activity but it is currently unclear how these affect the fragrance and flavor of the final beer (Steiner et al., 2012).

The manufacture of beer by partial or total substitution with adjuncts has been the subject of several investigations, with basic sensory evaluation of the adjunct-based brews. According to Kunz et al. (2012), adding up to 50% unmalted barley to the grain yielded a beer with preference ratings for flavor and odor equivalent to those of an all-malt beer. However, an increase in astringency was noted as the barley inclusion was raised to 90%. However, according to Steiner et al. (2012), the use of 100% unmalted barley has resulted in beers with less body and mouthfeel.

5.2 MAIZE

Drying reduces the moisture content of maize (corn), which is harvested with a water content of 25–30%. Crude fiber and inorganic materials are present in trace levels in maize's dry matter. The germ of the maize contains the oil. Maize is degermed before processing, effectively removing all oil because of worries about the oil's detrimental impact on foam. Degermed maize has an oil level of around 1%, while oil concentrations of up to 1.5% are also acceptable. The protein level drops to roughly 7–9% percent when the food is processed into grits or flakes. Because most of this protein does not dissolve during mashing, a lower protein content, corresponding to the maize fraction, must be anticipated. This may have an impact on the yeast's ability to obtain low-molecular-weight protein.

Even in terms of appearance, maize starch resembles barley starch. Furthermore, as maize starch gelatinizes at a temperature between 60 and 70°C, processing shouldn't present any difficulties. Degermed maize has a similar extract concentration as malt at 88–90% by dry weight.

Before processing, dried corn is degermed, with the husk and germ removed using a plan-sifter and aspirator. The following goods can be made from maize processing: grated corn, corn flakes, polished grits, and corn sugar.

5.3 CORN GRITS

Grits made from maize typically have a relatively big grain size (0.3–1.5 mm). A brewery's adjunct mill can be used for grinding. In an auxiliary cooker, corn grits are pretreated with roughly a fourth of the malt mash.

5.4 CORN FLAKES

Grits that have been slightly wet can be rolled into flat flakes and gelatinized in this way. The flakes can be mashed without first being treated with malt mash in this gelatinized state.

5.5 REFINED CORN GRITS

These are made by steeping grits in hot water at a temperature of 50°C (122°F) for 30 to 40 hours. The water is treated with SO_2 to kill off microorganisms. In a mill, the corn kernels are split open, and a separating mechanism removes the germ. Following the separation of the starch from the husk and protein, the crude starch is repeatedly washed before being dried. Outside the brewery, this procedure is carried out in specialized facilities. The manufactured maize starch is extremely finely split (0.5 mm average grain size). Due to the risk of a dust explosion posed by the refined corn grit's tiny particle size, they are delivered to the brewery in special trucks. As a result, refined corn grits are entirely made of malt starch, gelatinize quickly, and are simple to pour. Of the extract, 90–95% is in fat, ranging from 0.5 to 0.8%.

While adding maize can result in a fuller mouthfeel, using rice in the brewing process is thought to provide neutral, clean, and dry sensory qualities in the beer. However, there is a paucity of extensive sensory research evaluating the effects of employing high grist ratios of a variety of unmalted cereals, as well as complete sensory and analytical data about the flavor profile caused by adjuncts (Bogdan et al., 2017).

5.6 RICE

Broken rice, or grains that break during de-husking and polishing and, as a result, do not look as nice as unbroken grains, is used for brewing. Rice grains contain between 12 and 13% water. The dry substance contains around 85–90% starch, 5–8% protein, 0.2–0.4% oil, and small quantities of inorganic materials. The starch content of rice is made up of small distinct or aggregated granules with a distinctive form. The combined granules are made up of several component granules that are difficult to separate.

At temperatures between 70 and 85°C, rice starch expands significantly and gelatinizes. Higher gelatinization temperatures (80–85°C) are more common for some varieties of rice and rice that was harvested after experiencing hotter growing circumstances. When utilizing rice, this needs to be kept in mind. Because there is a low protein level and little of it dissolves during mashing, the malt mash must provide the free amino nitrogen (FAN) required by the yeast. In rice grits that have been formed by milling in a brewery and pretreated with some of the malt mash are crushed into rice flakes, becoming gelatinized as a result, and then fed directly to the mash tun.

Due to its expense, rice is currently mostly consumed in Asian nations. They employ broken grains, a by-product of rice cultivation for human use. De-husking and degerming must be done before continuing the processes. Typically, a variety mix is given, which causes a lot of variation in the temperature at which starch gelatinizes and the length of time that wort takes to separate. Beer is said to taste neutral, dry, light, and clean when rice is added. Corn results in a beer with a richer flavor. The oil-rich microorganisms in corn must be eliminated before it can be turned into grits or flakes for brewing (Yeo & Liu, 2014).

Because the used rice is de-husked and the used corn grits do not include husks, which act as a filter layer during lautering, there cannot be excessive amounts of rice or maize in the grist when a brewery utilizes a lauter tun. For wheat, which contains a lot of pentosans that make it more viscous, coarse grinding is advised to solve wort filtering issues. It is important to note that the quality requirements for raw barley used as an addition differ from those for barley used in the production of malt. The amount of protein in the grain must be high; the viability of the grain (germination energy and capacity) is unimportant.

5.7 BARLEY

The enzymes in malt can easily handle an adjunct of up to 15 to 20% barley. Milled barley or barley flakes that are formed from husked or de-husked barley can be used. The cheaper price relative to malt must be considered in addition to the decreased extract yield. Problems may arise when the a-glucan is not dissolved and is not properly broken down during mashing as a result of the lack of a malting procedure. Filtration issues are to be expected in such a situation.

Wet milling methods are advised for grinding since raw barley is a hard grain. Because unmalted barley has a high content of hemicelluloses and gums (10.3% DM), digesting it frequently necessitates adding exogenous hemicellulases to the mash (Annemuller & Manger, 2013). Rice and corn contain 2.3 and 4.2% DM of hemicellulose, respectively. During the malting process, hemicelluloses, which make up the majority of the cell walls in barley malt, are broken down. The fact that precooked adjuncts contain partially degraded hemicelluloses and gelatinized starch makes them easier to handle and provides more extract than raw ingredients. Even in infusion mashes, it is quite simple to process flaking rice or maize and produce high extracts. However, using these specific adjuncts at this time is not financially viable (Krottenthaler et al., 2009).

5.8 WHEAT

Wheat is frequently used in malted form, such as for making various kinds of wheat beers, although it is infrequently used as an unmalted auxiliary. Due to its high-extract yield, wheat malt often makes up between 50 and 60% of the ingredients needed to make wheat beers. There is still no specific brewing wheat variety since only a small portion of the wheat harvest is utilized for brewing. Great efforts have been made to grow brewing wheat strains in order to further enhance the quality of wheat beer. Winter-specific cultivars are preferred because of their reduced protein and increased extract content. They also provide a lighter beer.

The distinctive protein in wheat is called gluten. About 80% of the total protein is made up of a variety of distinct proteins, which mostly consist of glutelin and gliadin (instead of the hordein in barley). When wheat flour and water are mixed and kneaded, a sticky material forms that may be drawn into ropes and that, when dried, takes on the appearance of a horn. The high protein level in wheat makes it tough to process, which is unfavorable for the manufacture of brewing malt.

During threshing, wheat loses its husk and is afterwards "huskless." The increased viscosity of worts made from wheat malt is not a result of p-glucan but rather of pentosans.

5.9 MILLETS

Large-grained sorghum millet is a cereal that is mostly cultivated in the drier, hotter parts of Africa. In contrast, Europe cultivates small-grained millet for use as bird food. Only large-grained sorghum is utilized for making beer. Sorghum comes in a number of varieties, including spadix and panicle.

It is only logical that efforts to use the local raw material, sorghum, as a source of extract for beer production and to malt it are growing in many African nations in order to reduce the cost of expensive malt imports. Another factor is the unsuitability of the climate for growing brewing barley in many African nations. Sorghum develops enzymes as it grows, which can be utilized to dissolve the storage material it holds. However, sorghum has a lesser enzyme potential than barley.

Sorghum is cultivated and harvested throughout the wet season. Therefore, it is necessary to prepare for widespread contamination by microorganisms, especially fungus. In order to prevent spoiling, it is crucial to treat the harvested crop.

In these nations, breeding and cultivation of pure types are still in their infancy. Because the observed values are so disparate, it is hard to calculate averages.

Iodine-negative starch hydrolysates from corn, wheat, or rice can resemble malt worts in terms of their sugar content when made off-line by enzymatic and/or acid hydrolysis. These are made from the endosperm of grains after the germ and bran have been separated. Depending on the level of starch hydrolysis they have experienced, a broad range of syrups may also be utilized, each with a unique mix of fermentable (glucose, maltose, and maltotriose) and non-fermentable (maltotetraose and higher oligosaccharides) sugars. Although this does not give a complete picture of the sugar spectrum in the syrup and therefore of the fermentability of the supplemented wort, dextrose equivalent (DE) value, which corresponds to the percentage concentration of reducing sugars, is sometimes used to classify syrups. Syrups high in maltose are preferred over those high in glucose. Fermentation is slowed or stopped in worts with high glucose concentrations because yeasts find it difficult to adapt to metabolizing maltose and maltotriose. Large-scale brewers now frequently employ syrups made from starch. With no additional expenditure on the part of the brewery, syrups enable wort strength to be increased. Additionally, by guaranteeing the consistency of the wort and beer's composition, these adjuncts help solve the challenges caused by the heterogeneity of raw grains. They also lessen the amount of storage space needed for cereal raw ingredients. Utilizing syrups or sugar can result in material and energy cost benefits (Bogdan et al., 2017).

Exogenous enzymes are the sole way to attain good sorghum processability. Even with infusion mashing, brewing with up to 50% whole-grain sorghum flour is possible, but using sorghum grain necessitates pregelatinizing its starch through heating (Schnitzenbaumer et al., 2014). With more than 25% sorghum, it is difficult to separate the wort in the lauter tun, even with the use of commercial enzyme mixes. The enzyme activity of barley malt is adequate for digesting barley adjuncts in amounts less than 10–20%. To prevent lautering and filtering issues with larger amounts of barley adjuncts, microbial b-glucanase must be used. Exogenous proteinase is further needed at adjunct levels above 25%, while other enzymes, such as a-amylase, are required at adjunct levels over 50% (Annemuller & Manger, 2013). However, it has been claimed that using up to 50% of adjuncts and enzymes from barley during the brewing process can still result in beer with high attenuation and flavor stability (Kunz et al., 2012).

Mash vessel adjuncts include items that are not precooked but can be mixed directly with grist, like wheat flours; precooked outside the brewery, like flaked maize or rice grits, micronized and torrefied whole grains, flaked wheat or barley, and flaked pearl barley; and not precooked but can be mixed directly with grist, like cornmeal; grits; flours; and refined starches made from rice, maize, or sorghum that must be cooked in the brewery during mashing.

The varying gelatinization temperatures of starches generated from distinct sources are linked to this split. Before the adjunct starch can be combined with the malt mash, it must first undergo starch gelatinization because some adjunct starches, such as rice starch, gelatinize at temperatures higher than those at which malt enzymes are active.

If infusion mashing is used, this calls for a cereal cooker, an extra vessel in the brewhouse. It is recommended to utilize exogenous α-amylase or a fraction of highly enzymatic crushed malt when cooking grits, especially rice-based grits. Before the addition of the malt grits and water, uncooked cereals can also gelatinize in the mash vessel. However, this process delays wort production.

Infusion mashes can be made directly with wheat flour. However, the flour can be presoaked or precooked to get a greater extract, generally at 96°C to prevent foaming. Additionally, this guarantees that the little starch granules in it will gelatinize. Endosperm is the primary source of wheat flour. When the germ and bran are removed, the starch content rises, and the protein, ash, and fat levels fall, resulting in a greater extract yield. It can be challenging to work with flour, and it requires specific tools, including specialist hoppers and conveyers. As the chemical makeup of specific adjuncts differs, this affects the quality of beer. Understanding these relationships is crucial for modifying the manufacturing process, such as by choosing the best mashing profile or the proper enzymatic preparations (Bogdan et al., 2017).

The kind and quality of the adjunct, the pretreatment technique, the use of enzymatic preparations, the quality of the malt, the mashing operation, and the wort separation system are just a few of the variables that affect the amount of mash vessel adjuncts in the grist. To shorten the time needed for wort separation when using a lot of grain adjuncts, mash filters are advised. The percentage of maize or rice grits in the grist shouldn't be more than 30 to 40% if no enzyme preparations were used during the mashing process. Malt substitution levels greater than 40% require the use of α-amylase (Cooper et al., 2016). However, it might be challenging to separate the wort in the lauter tun with such grist mixes.

Without the use of exogenous enzymes, processing oats up to 20% allows for the creation of high-quality wort (Schnitzenbaumer et al., 2014). Without using exogenous enzymes, it is even possible to make respectable beers with up to 40% oats, but only if the oats are hammer milled. But substituting hammer-milled oats for 20–40% of the barley malt results in a large rise in the mash's β-glucan content and a significant drop in the filtration/lautering rate.

Sensory evaluation of the beers brewed with unmalted barley, rice, corn, and wheat adjuncts is important. In order to comprehend the underlying causes of the sensory qualities of adjunct beers, it is also important to grasp the chemical makeup of each beer.

5.10 MALT EXTRACTS

Malt extracts are a favorite among homebrewers and microbreweries. They can be purchased both hopped and unhopped. The final wort can be supplemented with liquid

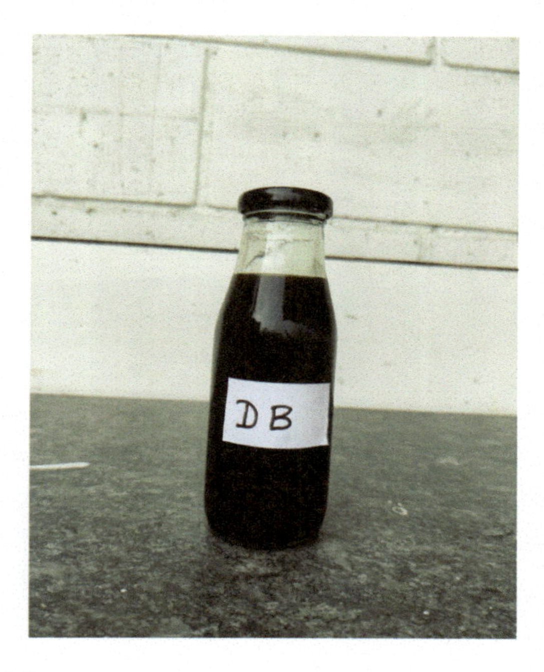

FIGURE 5.1 Dark Beer

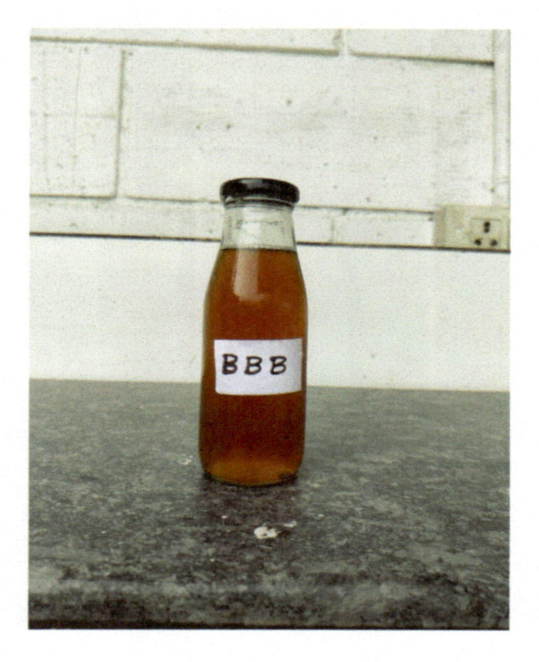

FIGURE 5.2 Blueberry Beer

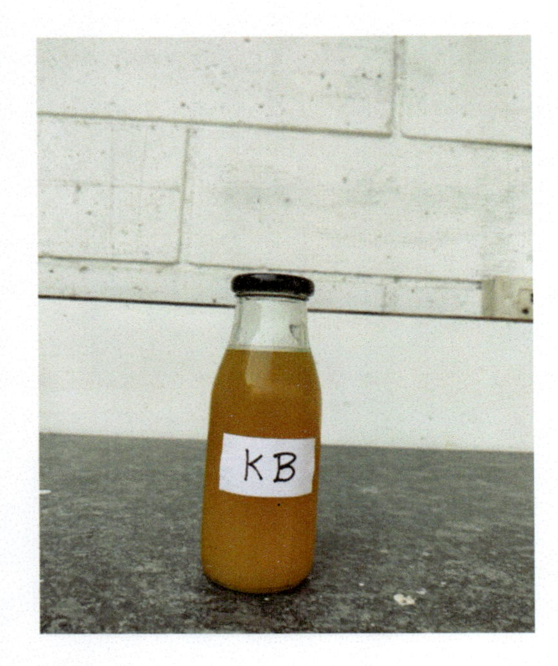

FIGURE 5.3 Kinnow Beer

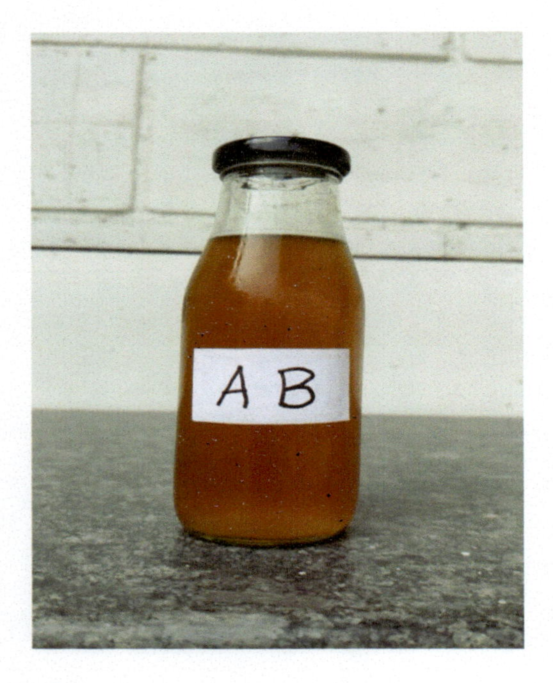

FIGURE 5.4 Amber Beer

adjuncts and granulated sugar, both of which contain soluble sugars. As a result, they are referred to as copper or kettle adjuncts. These are frequently employed to create high-gravity worts, which serve to enhance the brewhouse's capacity and, as a result, the brewery's overall output. Sucrose is employed in both solid and liquid forms as disaccharides or inverted sugar following hydrolysis, allowing for simple adjustment of wort fermentability (a mixture of glucose and fructose). However, concentrated sugar solutions have a tendency to crystallize, necessitating heated handling and storage at 40–50°C (Bogdan et al., 2017).

5.11 SUGAR OR SUGAR SYRUP

Cane sugar or beet sugar (saccharose) may be substituted for some of the grain load in the brewing of beer that has not been brewed in accordance with the Purity Law. A disaccharide comprising glucose and fructose is called saccharose. The saccharose is inverted into the two monosaccharides and then becomes easily fermentable if boiling is prolonged or acid is introduced. Since the sugar is totally fermentable and needs no prior preparation, it is added to the casting wort.

Sugar's solubility is its most crucial quality. There is a particularly high level of sugar solubility in water; 100 parts water and 204 parts sugar dissolve at 20°C. Much more saccharose dissolves in hot water, but it precipitates back out as it cools. At least 65% of produced sugar syrup is sugar. This allows for simple storage and prevents microorganism assault since they plasmolyze in the high-percentage solution. The solution's high pressure forces the water out of the microorganisms' cells. Since a syrup solution cannot deteriorate, if the solution is not sterilized, the microorganisms will quickly reactivate in a diluted condition.

The sugar is usually dissolved cold but occasionally hot, which requires more energy. It is typically purchased in a dissolved state, and classifications are made between liquid sugar with a sugar content of approximately 65%, a non-inverted saccharose solution with a maximum of 3% inverted sugar, inverted liquid sugar with a rate of inversion less than 50%, and inverted sugar with a rate of inversion greater than 50%.

Liquid sugar is typically utilized in the brewing of beer since inversion happens naturally when wort boils. The flavor of beer is not negatively impacted by small amounts of added sugar since it has gone through full fermentation. However, it must be remembered that sugar does not provide any nitrogen molecules to the wort; therefore, the nitrogen level of the amino acids may be too low, which may cause fermentation issues. If an affordable source of sugar is available, including liquid sugar as an extract supplier simply makes sense.

When sugar is melted or sugar syrup is heated, brown products with a familiar caramel flavor are created. Depending on the pH level, this procedure may be more focused on producing colors (such as couleur) or aromas. Many aroma compounds are produced when saccharose syrup is cooked in a buffered solution (dihydro furanone, cyclopentenolone, and others). In the case of caramelized brewing sugar, this is intended. It is necessary to keep a watchful eye on any potential carcinogenic acryia mide development. Brewing sugar that has been caramelized is offered for sale as syrup or brown sugar.

Undried refined maize grits in which the starch has been hydrolyzed to sugar are used to make glucose syrup (i.e. splitting with water). For this, three procedures are employed: combining enzymatic hydrolysis with acid hydrolysis using enzyme hydrolysis.

Starch, including amylopectin and amylose, is composed of lengthy chains of glucose residues. When an acid is supplied, a water molecule is inserted, breaking the bonds between the glucose molecules, resulting in the production of glucose. The bonds are gradually broken during this procedure, which involves adding diluted hydrochloric acid (0.10 to 0.15%), heating, and pressure. As a consequence, a syrup made of sugar and dextrins is created. Centrifugation is used to eliminate any soluble components, and the syrup is then concentrated to around 60%.

A greater amount of glucose and maltose can be obtained if the breakdown is carried out in conjunction with an enzymatic treatment or with enzymes alone, and this results in a noticeably superior extract composition for fermentation. The glucose syrup's composition is flexible within large bounds. A term Dextrose equivalent used to indicate the degree of hydrolysis of starch into glucose. It is the percentage of the total solids that have been converted to reducing sugars: the higher the DE, the more sugars and less dextrins are present.

The mash can be thinner when syrups or sugar are employed, which makes it simpler to extract and separate the wort from raw components. There is also less contamination of yeast cells during fermentation as a result of the decreased levels of sludge in pitching wort.

5.12 REFERENCES

Annemuller, G., & Manger, H. J. (2013). *Processing of various adjuncts in beer production* (1st ed.). VLB.

Bogdan, P., & Kordialik-Bogacka, E. (2017). Alternatives to malt in brewing. *Trends in Food Science and Technology*, *65*, 1–9.

Cooper, C. M., Evans, D. E., Yousif, A., Metz, N., & Koutoulis, A. (2016). Comparison of the impact on the performance of small-scale mashing with different proportions of unmalted barley, Ondea Pro®, malt and rice. *Journal of the Institute of Brewing*, *122*(2), 218–227.

Goode, D. L., Wijngaard, H. H., & Arendt, E. K. (2005). Mashing with unmalted barley-impact of malted barley and commercial enzyme (Bacillus spp.) additions. *Technical Quarterly-Master Brewers Association of the Americas*, *42*(3), 184–198.

Habschied, K., Zivkovic, A., Krstanovic, V., & Mastanjevic, K. (2020). Functional beer-A review on possibilities. *Beverages*, *6*(3), 51.

Kok, Y., Ye, L., Muller, J., Ow, D., & Bi, X. (2019). Brewing with malted barley or raw barley: What makes the difference in the processes? *Applied Microbiology and Biotechnology*, *103*, 1059–1067.

Krottenthaler, M., Back, W., & Zarnkow, M. (2009). Wort production. In *Handbook of brewing: Processes, technology, markets*, Willey-VCH (pp. 165–205).

Kunz, T., Muller, C., Mato-Gonzales, D., & Methner, F. J. (2012). The influence of unmalted barley on the oxidative stability of wort and beer. *Journal of the Institute of Brewing*, *118*, 32–39.

Li, X., Takahashi, T., Suzuki, N., & Kaiser, H. M. (2011). The impact of climate change on maize yields in the United States and China. *Agricultural Systems*, *104*, 348–353.

Schnitzenbaumer, B., Kaspar, J., Titze, J., & Arendt, E. K. (2014). Implementation of commercial oat and sorghum flours in brewing. *European Food Research and Technology, 238*, 515–525.

Steiner, E., Auer, A., Becker, T., & Gastl, M. (2012). Comparison of beer quality attributes between beers brewed with 100% barley malt and 100% barley raw material. *Journal of the Science of Food and Agriculture, 92*, 803–813.

Xie, W., Xiong, W., Pan, J., Ali, T., Cui, Q., Guan, D., Meng, J., Mueller, N. D., Lin, E., & Davis, S. J. (2018). Decreases in global beer supply due to extreme drought and heat. *Nature Plants, 4*, 964–973.

Yeo, H. Q., & Liu, S. Q. (2014). An overview of selected specialty beers: Developments, challenges and prospects. *Journal of Food Science and Technology, 49*, 1607–1618.

Yorke, J., Cook, D., & Ford, R. (2021). Brewing with unmalted cereal adjuncts: Sensory and analytical impacts on beer quality. *Beverages, 7*(1), 4.

6 Role of Temperature in Brewing

Brewing is a centuries-old craft with evidence from many significant civilizations throughout history, dating back thousands of years. This heritage is now more of a science than an art because of technology. Prior to the development of the steam engine, thermometers, and other pieces of technology, the majority of beer was produced on a relatively small scale, with a great deal of inconsistency and unfavorable tastes. Recipes changed according to families, ingredients, climate, and geographic regions. Brewing evolved into a craft that has been honed over centuries utilizing antiquated methods that could only be learned via experience and trial and error. A beer that was produced using techniques and temperature control throughout the fermentation cooling process was very different from the ales that are currently popular in the United States.

Due to the increasing popularity of and desire for small-batch brews, modern brewing has experienced its own revolution. Over the past few years, microbreweries and home breweries have grown. Breweries may now make beer the old-fashioned way, but with a modern twist, thanks to the process cooling equipment that is becoming more widely available and less expensive.

The most important control in the brewing process is temperature, both hot and cold. Temperature control is critical throughout the brewing process, especially during the mash, to ensure that complex sugars are converted to fermentable sugars that can later be fermented by yeast. During fermentation, temperature control is critical to ensure proper yeast performance as well as to control the production of secondary flavor and aroma compounds produced by yeast metabolism. Because this is such an important step in making great beer, every brewery must maintain strict control.

6.1 TYPES OF TEMPERATURE MEASUREMENTS IN BREWING

6.1.1 Spot Measurements

Spot measurements are periodic checks to make sure the beer's temperature is within the right range. This is a crucial quality-auditing tool for checking the efficiency of temperature-controlled processes by taking a random measurement of them.

6.1.2 Point Measurements

When it is necessary to reach a specific objective, such with sparge water temperature in the brewery, point measurements are helpful. The temperature gauges will need to be quick and accurate in order to be certain that the information they are

DOI: 10.1201/b22906-6

providing is correct. Since these measurements frequently focus on a range rather than a precise temperature, they must be accurate to +/–1°C.

6.1.3 Constant Measurement

Fermentation and mashing are the two main stages of the brewing process at which continuous temperature measuring takes place. In order to activate the enzymes required for the conversion of starches into fermentable sugar by way of α- and β-amylases and to avoid exceeding the denaturation point for these enzymes, saccharification must be obtained when mashing. Because α-amylase functions best between 70–75°C (158–167°F) and denatures beyond 80°C (176°F), β-amylase is most active between 60–65°C (140–149°F). Practically, the majority of brewers use a temperature range between 62–75°C (145–158°F), depending on the desired level of β- or α-amylase activity. Due to the relative narrowness of this range, it is essential to be able to assess and regulate these temperatures within a constrained range; otherwise, the danger of producing unfermentable wort exists.

Fermentation is the second important area that requires ongoing observation. In order to maintain constant performance and secondary flavor and aroma ingredients, yeast is very dependent on appropriate fermentation temperatures. Even a little variation in temperature, especially early in the fermentation process, can significantly influence the formation of ester and fusel (higher) alcohol molecules and radically alter the sensory characteristics of the beer. Additionally, temperatures during later phases of fermentation will affect overall beer quality: for example, crashing beer to remove yeast from suspension or raising the temperature of lager fermentation by a few degrees for diacetyl rest. At this point, maintaining rigorous temperature control is crucial, and to maintain the most efficient regulation, glycol (or other temperature factors) must be kept within +/–0.5°F.

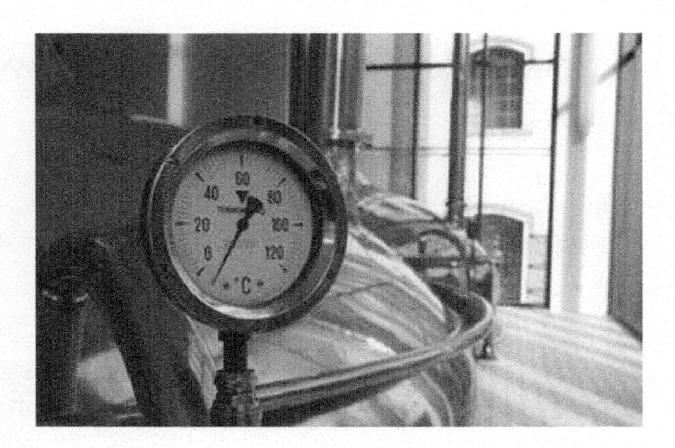

FIGURE 6.1 Temperature Gauge

6.2 TEMPERATURE GAUGE

Much like cooking, brewing requires a "feel" for the art, but there are still crucial foundational principles that must be followed. One of the foundations that can really make or break beer is temperature management, which is also one of the simplest to handle with a few basic instruments. The temperature gauge is an important piece of brewhouse equipment.

6.3 TEMPERATURE AT VARIOUS BREWING STEPS

Each and every step of brewing is temperature controlled and monitored. While temperature monitoring is critical during the mashing process, it should not be overlooked during storage or serving. Warm lagers or overly chilled stouts are simply unpalatable.

6.4 MASHING

The hot water steeping process that hydrates the grains and activates the malt enzymes that convert the grain starches into fermentable sugars is known as mashing in brewing. The final beer has different outcomes and flavor profiles depending on the mashing temperature. Temperature control during mashing is very important.

There are numerous enzymes in the mash that require a specific temperature and pH range to function optimally. During the mash, enzymes work to break down complex sugars and make them available for the yeast to consume during fermentation.

Enzymes in the mash are responsible not only for starch conversion but also for lowering pH, breaking down gums and proteins, and producing yeast nutrients. There are also enzymes that convert starches to various sugars, some of which are more fermentable than others. Because each enzyme performs a different function, the sugar profile in the wort will vary depending on the mash conditions (temperature and pH).

During mashing, once the enzymes present in the barley are activated, they start the conversion of starch to sugar. Brewers can control the types of sugars produced by changing the water temperature, which is usually between 37 and 76°C.

Lower mash temperatures create highly fermentable sugar, which makes a beer with a dry finish. Keeping the mash temperature too low (below 140°F) for too long results in a "watery" beer that doesn't taste good. Some unfermented sugars are also desired to produce a sweeter, full-bodied beer. This is accomplished by increasing the temperature of the water, which makes sugars more difficult for yeast to digest (Muller, 1991).

Starch conversion will halt or slow down if the mash is heated to a temperature above 75–76°C (168–170°F). Fortunately, enzymes are not quickly destroyed at high temperatures. It would take around ten minutes to "mash out" the enzymes in an attempt to destroy (denature) them. Tannin extraction from the grain husks is a danger when mashing or sparging at or above 76°C (170°F). Beer becomes astringent when the tannins are removed, and this characteristic does not usually change as the beer ages. Astringency is an unpleasant flavor that tastes like a combination of dryness and bitterness; it tastes like a teabag.

TABLE 6.1
Major Mashing Enzymes, Optimum Temperature, Optimum pH, and Their Functions

Enzyme	Optimum Temperature Range	Optimum pH	Function
Phytase	86–126°F (30–52°C)	5.0–5.5	Also called the "acid rest," it was used to lower the mash's pH, but it has been discontinued with the proper use of water chemistry.
Debranching	95–113°F (35–45°C)	5.0–5.8	Helps increase the solubility of starches resulting in increased extraction of certain malts. This enzyme breaks down the 1–6 links in starches.
β-Glucanase	95–113°F (35–45°C)	4.5–5.5	Working within the same temperature range as debranching, this enzyme is best at breaking down gums.
Protease	113–131°F (45–55°C)	4.6–5.3	This protein rest breaks up large proteins that form haze.
Peptidase	113–131°F (45–55°C)	4.6–5.3	Peptidase breaks down the smaller amino acid chains released by proteinase but only works from the ends, releasing yeast nutrients such as free amino nitrogen (FAN).
β-Amylase	131–150°F (55–66°C)	5.0–5.5	The final enzymatic process involves the conversion of starches into dextrins and fermentable sugars. The starches must be gelatinized for this to take place.
α-Amylase	154–162°F (68–72°C)	5.3–5.7	Temperatures above 155°F favor this enzyme, producing a more dextrinous wort, which is less fermentable and results in a fuller body.

6.5 MAJOR MASH ENZYMES

In some cases, mashing is also done at 67°C (152°F). At this temperature, both β- and α-amylase enzymes work, extracting the highest amount of fermentable sugars.

6.6 PROTEIN REST

Holding mash at 35–45°C (95–115°F) for 20 to 30 minutes is called protein rest of mash. This step is necessary in case of moderately modified malt (like some European malts), mash, or if there is 20% or more β-glucan–containing adjuncts in the mash. At this temperature, the enzyme phytase acidifies the mash, lowering the pH.

6.7 SACCHARIFICATION REST

The most crucial stage of mashing is a rest at a temperature at which both α- and β-amylase function and create a wort that is packed with sugars that yeast can ferment. The 60–70°C temperature range is a compromise between the two enzymes. Both α- and β-amylase are capable of breaking down the bigger carbohydrates.

A wort that is lighter in body and more fermentable will produce at a peak performance at 65°C, leading to increased attenuation (also depending on the yeast). Therefore, if a drier beer with less residual sugars or dextrins is preferred, use the lower mash temperature.

The β-amylase will quickly deteriorate past 65°C and cease to function, but will still retain α-amylase. As a result, the wort will have more residual sugar, giving the beer a sweeter finish and a fuller body.

The mash temperature is also responsible for the development of a good foam quality in beer. The proteins in the finished beer are influenced by the temperature at which the mash is conducted.

For foam stability, the protein and lipid composition of the finished product is essential. Most proteins are foam promoters, meaning they aid in the creation of a more stable head. Lipids, on the other hand, can rapidly reduce the stability of foam. At temperatures below 55°C, proteins that promote foam are neutralized, and as temperatures rise, their concentrations grow as well. At temperatures below 55°C, enzymes that support fatty acids, which undermine foam stability, become active.

6.8 FERMENTATION TEMPERATURE

No matter when or where beer is brewed, fermentation is always essential to success. Yeast converts the glucose in wort into ethyl alcohol and carbon dioxide during fermentation. Beer's alcohol level and carbonation are both a result of this.

Temperature, the kind of yeast used (liquid or dry), and the type of beer (lager or ale) are all related to the fermentation process. When dry yeast is used, beer fermentation usually takes 1–3 days and when liquid yeast is used, beer ferments in around 8–14 days. Lagers ferment at a lower temperature; therefore, the process usually takes two weeks or longer.

Temperature is a crucial consideration during the fermentation process. The ideal range for ale fermentation is 18–22°C. Lower temperatures, between 10–12°C, are needed for lager. When fermentation occurs above these optimal temperature limits, harsh-tasting fusel alcohols and very fruity-flavored esters are produced.

The fermentation process may completely halt if the temperature becomes too high. It's crucial, but challenging, to maintain the correct temperature range for ale or lager. Even at ideal environmental temperatures, the heat produced by the fermentation process can raise the temperature.

Beer aroma is also known to be influenced by fermentation temperature. Low-temperature fermentation is said to produce beer with better flavor and fragrance as well as higher levels of ethanol and beer yield. Nevertheless, breweries employ high-gravity worts and ferment at higher temperatures in an effort to conserve energy, space, and time. To achieve the appropriate alcohol concentration, the product is diluted with deaerated water after fermentation (Kucharczyk & Tuszynski, 2018).

6.9 CONTROL OF FERMENTATION TEMPERATURE

The majority of beers were traditionally made during the cooler months and kept in basements or caves to preserve the right temperatures. Today, however, there are a number of procedures that can maintain the ideal temperature for brews all year round.

Fermenters usually have triple jackets. The outermost jacket is for insulation purposes, and prevents evaporation and helps maintain the temperature of the fermenters.

The second or middle jacket is for chilling media. Chilling media are usually glycol or chilled water, which circulates through the middle jacket to maintain the desired temperature. Flow is maintained by automation valves controlled by the sensors installed for fermenter temperature, so chilling media will circulate whenever it is required. Middle jackets are usually dimple or coil shaped. The innermost jacket of the tank contains the beer.

In places where the temperature is too low or in cold conditions, the temperature of fermentation tanks is maintained by using hot water. Hot water is circulated through the middle jacket instead chilling media, which works same way as chilling media but will raise the temperature.

The average ale yeast works best between 18–22°C. This is the ideal range for yeast to ferment without giving off too many undesirable flavors. Warmer temperatures make yeast thrive, but they also speed up reproduction and increase the production of esters. By pitching enough yeast and regulating the temperature, this can be prevented.

Fusel alcohols: Often said to have a hot, almost drunken or vodka-like alcohol flavor This usually diminishes throughout conditioning.

Esters: Frequently associated with fruity flavors like banana, pear, or nail polish remover. While certain esters are nice in some beer varieties, such as hefeweizens, they frequently punch you in the face when they shouldn't. Esters can decrease while you're training, but high quantities might never improve.

Acetaldehyde: This substance is frequently associated with green apples, raw pumpkin or squash, or Jolly Ranchers. Every fermentation produces acetaldehyde as a natural by-product; nevertheless, under unregulated circumstances, it can accumulate excessively.

Each of previously mentioned off-flavors are quite normal and will manifest to varying degrees in every fermentation. Simply said, they are harder to find in the best fermentation circumstances.

6.10 IDEAL YEAST-PITCHING TEMPERATURE

Yeast-pitching temperature is also a crucial point. Pitching at cooler temperatures is the right way because it gives an environment to yeast to grow during fermentation. In the fermenter, the temperature rises throughout fermentation (controlled by the chilling system), so fermentation will begin at a low temperature.

6.11 TYPES OF YEAST

6.11.1 Ale

Ale yeasts are top-fermenting yeasts with a wide temperature range in which they can ferment. It was often observed that a good pale ale or a superb IPA is best fermenter at 18–22°C. Warmer brewing techniques can enhance the banana and clove flavors that are typical of German-style wheat beers. In case of German wheat beers, if fermentation is carried out below 20°C, then the clove flavor will be enhanced, and above 20°C, the banana flavor will be more prominent. Similar to this, saison beers can be fermented at a temperature around 20°C to provide more of the fruitiness and spice than anticipated from a Belgian saison.

6.11.2 Lager

Lager yeasts are bottom-fermenting yeasts that brew cleanest when the temperature is lower. These yeasts give excellent lagers and pilsners their crispness. While several lager yeasts have optimal brewing temperatures between 10 and 14°C, most do so in this range. Many brewers choose to brew their lagers in the winter because of this lower temperature range since it works with seasonal temperatures.

6.11.3 Hybrid Yeasts

While the characteristics of ale and lager yeasts are quite obvious, some strains exhibit traits from both. Even though California lager yeast is a lager yeast, it brews best at ale temperatures. These yeasts imitate the crispness of lager while brewing at 18 to 20°C, although they are not a replacement for an excellent lager yeast.

6.11.4 New Kveik Yeasts

These yeasts with Norwegian origins brew hotter and more quickly than conventional strains. This category has a variety of strains, some of which ferment cleanly and others that are better suited for farmhouse ales. The Voss strain, which ferments with a clear flavor in its optimal temperature range of 30–35°C, is one of the most popular strains. In addition, fermentation normally completes in three to four days at these temperatures.

High temperatures, high yeast-pitching rates, and high wort gravities are frequent practical techniques to fermentation intensification (Brown & Hammond, 2003). By encouraging yeast growth, higher temperatures and faster pitching rates accelerate the process of fermentation. These simple methods, however, have a number of drawbacks, such as changed beer flavor at the conclusion of primary fermentation and harmful effects on yeast viability and vitality, resulting in subsequent fermentation performance (Lekkas et al., 2005).

The range of 8–16°C is the ideal temperature for bottom fermentation. Increased yeast activity, worsened foam stability, worsened beer color, decreased pH, and greater loss of bitter chemicals might all result from increased temperature in bottom fermentation. For fermentation to proceed at an optimum rate, the weight of the extract should not decrease more than 1.5% in 24 hours. For fermentation to continue, the temperature shouldn't drop more than 1°C in a 24-hour period (Basarova et al., 2010; Solgajova et al., 2013).

In actuality, one of the most useful tools for modifying fermentation pace is temperature management. If the temperature is raised from 10 to 13°C and then tempered to 14°C during the last stage of fermentation, the process might be sped up by roughly 28.8 hours (Sepelova, 2004). Even the sensory qualities of beer are improved by this alteration.

Wort has to have a sufficient amount of nutrients for yeast to survive and flourish. A supply of fermentable carbohydrates, assimilable nitrogen, molecular oxygen, the vitamin biotin, phosphorus and sulphur, calcium and magnesium ions, and trace minerals like copper and zinc are all necessary for yeast growth (Lewis & Young, 2002).

6.12 MATURATION TEMPERATURE

Between the conclusion of primary fermentation and the removal of yeast from the beer in order to prepare it for packing, there is a period called maturation. The majority of beers are not yet ready to drink when the yeast has finished its main task of metabolizing carbohydrates, even though most beer fermentation are technically finished in three to ten days. This is due to the fact that fermentation frequently results in characteristics that are deemed unpleasant in final beers. Because of this, beer has to mature in some way in order to taste good. Conditioning, lagering, and ageing are some other names for maturation.

Although fermentation and maturation are seen as different processes in conventional brewing techniques, they really have a lot of similarities. Many of the biological, physiological, and physical processes that take place during maturation are still poorly understood and explained.

At the conclusion of primary fermentation, vicinal diketones, hydrogen sulfide, and acetaldehyde are chiefly responsible for unfavorable tastes. Examples include the buttery-tasting diacetyl and the honey-like pentanedione. Because immature beer occasionally smells like green apples due to high acetaldehyde levels, it is frequently referred to as "green beer." All these unwanted chemicals undergo reduction throughout maturity, either via the continued work of the yeast or through other organic chemical routes.

Lager beers are moved into a different vessel, where leftover sugars (maltotriose and sometimes maltose) are gently fermented, after primary fermentation and chilling to around 0–4°C). As the yeast continues to release carbon dioxide, off tastes are diminished, and the beer becomes carbonated. Before the beer is put into a lagering (cold storage) vessel, krausening, the addition of a tiny part of fermenting beer, is occasionally carried out. Active yeast can be added at this stage to accelerate the beer's maturation and boost its natural carbonation.

The requirement for the many weeks of cold maturation known as "lagering" comes from the fact that cold-fermented beers tend to exhibit more "green" characteristics after the conclusion of primary fermentation than warm-fermented beers do.

Traditional methods for conditioning ales involve keeping the brew reasonably warm, often between 10 and 20°C (50 and 68°F). This storage duration can be fairly short because most ale yeasts respond quickly to warm temperatures, and many warm-fermented beers are ready for packaging within 14 days of brewing. In the UK, classic cask-conditioned ales are aged (conditioned) unfiltered in the barrel in the basement of the bar or public house.

A mild natural carbonation is added to the beer by the cask's ongoing fermentation. Prior to serving, the beer is clarified by using isinglass (collagen) to adsorb the yeast and other solid components (protein-polyphenol complexes) and settle them to the bottom of the barrel. Beers that are bottle-conditioned go through a second fermentation within the bottle. Although this results in carbonation, these beers often need to mature for a longer period of time in the bottle before being made available for sale.

Many brewers now ferment and mature beer in the cylindrical containers often referred to as unitanks since using secondary maturation vessels can be costly and labor intensive. By using their own cooling jackets, these tanks eliminate the need to transfer beer into a different container in a frigid cellar. The tanks' cone-shaped bottoms make it simple to remove the yeast that has accumulated as sediment.

Numerous attempts have been made to create continuous systems for the brewing process, including continuous maturation, by big breweries. Immobilized yeast cells have been used to create a continuous maturation process that speeds up beer ageing. On DEAE cellulose or glass beads, yeast cells are immobilized. By centrifuging the original fermentation yeast, diacetyl in the immature beer is quickly reduced. This young beer that has been clarified is heated to 90°C (194°F) for seven to eight minutes to completely transform all the precursor (α- acetolactate) into diacetyl. To avoid oxygen intake, care must be exercised.

After being heated, the beer is chilled again before being poured gently down a packed bed column of yeast cells that have been immobilized. Buttery diacetyl is transformed by these yeast cells into flavorless acetoin and butanediol. Other taste maturation processes also take place in a succession of unclear responses. Brewers disagree on whether this method results in beer of the finest quality, but it does shorten maturing durations from a few weeks to just two hours. A few sizable brewers only employ their immobilized yeast systems in the hot summer months when business is brisk. This process allows for the production of lager beer that is suitable for sale in as little as 10 days.

6.13 BEER-SERVING TEMPERATURE

Not all beers should be served extremely cold. The optimal temperature for each type of beer depends on its specific flavor profile. Most beer consumers aren't always aware of how much temperature affects a beer's ability to convey its character and flavors.

Most brews can't fully expose their qualities if they're served too cold; yeast esters are stifled and never fully develop, and the subtleties of hops' scent don't emerge as they should. In essence, the drinker is unable to taste or smell all the components intended for sensory perception. Despite the enormous shift towards delicious beer in the United States, which is evident in the recent growth of the craft beer business, it appears that the significance of beer-serving temperature is not completely appreciated.

Beer may be served at a range of temperatures, from several degrees above freezing to slightly below room temperature in a cool basement (considered warm). Each type has a perfect range that accentuates its unique qualities and encourages optimum pleasure.

Overall, extreme cold obscures tastes and heightens the bitterness, dryness, and carbonation of a beer. There isn't much to be gained from freezing a beer this far unless the intention is to mask its flavorless nature by enhancing the tickle of its effervescence (commonly the case with mass-market lagers).

The aromatic chemicals in a brew are aided in their release by heat and evaporation. Additionally, a beer tastes considerably better when its volatile organic chemicals are active since flavor is mostly impacted by our sense of smell (particularly retro-nasal olfaction).

For instance, it's thought that 5–6°C is the optimum temperature for a fine German pilsner's famous Saaz hop flavors and malt qualities to emerge. However, even at this low temperature, the style's sharp carbonation adds to a crisp drinking experience.

It is increasingly crucial for the whole spectrum of a beer's chemical components to emerge as the beverage becomes richer and heavier in the mouth. As a general rule, light-bodied beers with lower alcohol content taste better when served cold, whereas full-bodied beers with greater alcohol content benefit from being served somewhat warmer.

Beer-serving temperatures for different styles of beers include:

- At 1–4°C (very cold), mass-produced light lagers, malt liquor, and bottom-shelf beers are served.
- At 4–7°C (cold), wheat beers (such as Hefeweizen, Witbier, Gose, and Berliner Weisse), Czech and German pilsners, Munich Helles, and craft lagers are served.
- At 7–10°C (cool), IPAs, American pale ales, porters, most stouts, Munich and Franconian *dunkel* lagers, and amber lagers (Marzen) are served.
- At 10–13°C (cellar temperature), German Bock and Maibock lagers, most Belgian ales including saisons, sour ales, English bitter, English mild, Scottish ales, and Baltic porter are served.
- At 13–16°C (warm), strong, rich ales such as barley wine, double IPA, imperial stout, Belgian strong, and strong lagers such as German doppelbock are served.

Poured beer quickly loses carbonation; this is the major justification for serving mass-produced lagers ice cold. Low temperatures heighten the iconic tingling carbonation experience. The benefits of effervescence can no longer mask the apparent lack of taste when the beer warms and flattens.

Freezing glassware to keep a beer colder for a longer period of time frequently results in the glassware absorbing bad freezer aromas, which can have a negative effect on the drinking experience. Additionally, when the beer is poured, the ice crystals that have accumulated on the glass's surface prevent appropriate foam production.

A large German-style glass (mass) will work if you pour a beer that will be simple to drink and appreciated cold, such a Munich Helles or an American craft lager, and drink it quickly. A half-liter or pint glass is better for more deliberate consumption because the beer won't get too warm throughout the course of the drinking.

To counteract the unavoidable warming caused by the touch of the hands on the glass, attempt to serve beer just a little bit cooler than the style's ideal temperature. Simply hold the glass between your hands for a short period of time and gently swirl it to help the beer achieve the correct temperature if you are offered an excessively cold imperial stout, for example. Serve strong beer in properly stemmed smaller glasses since they may easily get overly warm if held and drunk over an extended period of time and are especially rich in alcohol when served warm.

6.14 REFERENCES

Basarova, G., Savel, J., Basar, P., & Lejsek, T. (2010). *Brewing: Theory and practice of beer production*. Publishing House UCT Prague.

Brown, A. K., & Hammond, J. R. M. (2003). Flavour control in small-scale beer fermentations. *Food and Bioproducts Processing*, *81*(1), 40–49.

Kucharczyk, K., & Tuszynski, T. (2018). The effect of temperature on fermentation and beer volatiles at an industrial scale. *Journal of the Institute of Brewing*, *124*(3), 230–235.

Lekkas, C., Stewart, G. G., Hill, A., Taidi, B., & Hodgson, J. (2005). The importance of free amino nitrogen in wort and beer. *Technical Quarterly-Master Brewers Association of the Americas, 42(2)*, 113.

Lewis, M. J., & Young, T. W. (2002). *Brewing*. Springer Science & Business Media.

Muller, R. (1991). The effects of mashing temperature and mash thickness on wort carbohydrate composition. *Journal of the Institute of Brewing*, *97*(2), 85–92.

Sepelova, G., Cvengroschova, M., & Smogrovicova, D. (2004). Temperature influence on fermentation speed and organoleptic beer properties. *Kvasny Prumysl*, 2, 41–42.

Solgajova, M., Francakova, H., Drab, S., & Toth, Z. (2013). Effect of temperature on the process of beer primary fermentation. *Journal of Microbiology, Biotechnology and Food Sciences*, 1791–1799.

7 Selective Improvisation of Beers

Beer is such a nice product that it may be nicely combined with different flavors, aromatic herbs, medicinal extracts, honey, sugar, coffee, and others. It may also be combined with several fruits like sweet fruit such as cherries, wild plums, and raspberries. This tradition of combining beer with different supplements dates back to the earliest period when the main objective was to get a beverage with unique and distinctive characteristics and mask deficiencies caused by inadequate production conditions (Dordevic et al., 2015).

7.1 BEERS HAVING FRUITS

Herbal extracts', fruits', and mushrooms' addition as adjuncts in beers was studied. These were usually added during the wort boiling, fermentation, maturation, and packaging stages. In some cases, the wort-boiling step is best, especially in case of herbs. The addition of fruits led to an increase in the beer's volatile profile and also an increase in sensory acceptability (Paiva et al., 2021).

Very promising research regarding fruit additions to beer concerns the addition of grapes. This combines the different bioactive compounds originating from wine and beer, primarily phenolic compounds and anthocyanins. Several research papers combining beer and wine have been published (Habschied et al., 2020).

In the last decade, the demand for special beers with improved healthy function has significantly increased, with or without new tastes. One of the possible mixes is beer with the bioactive components present in grapes that are responsible for the health-promoting functions of red wine. Veljovic et al. (2015) studied the effects of the addition of the Prokupac grape on the physicochemical properties, the fermentation kinetics of the grape beer were studied, and the results were compared with a control lager beer. The activity of yeast upon the addition of grapes was also studied. They observed that original extract, fermentation rate, alcohol content, and yeast growth were significantly higher in beers having grapes because of the presence of a higher concentration of simple sugars in grapes compared to pure wort. The color of beer samples based on the CIELAB chromatic parameters was observed, and the beer samples with grapes were yellow with a certain proportion of redness while the control beer was pure yellow. There was a reduction in the lightness and yellowness of beers with the increase in the concentration of grape while the redness of the samples was directly proportional to grape quantity. The phenolic content and antioxidant capacity of grape beers were significantly higher than those of the control beer, which indicates that grape beer is a better source of natural antioxidants than regular lager beer.

DOI: 10.1201/b22906-7

Another special beer was produced by fermenting wort combined with a must of Prokupac and Muscat Hamburg in different ratios. It was observed that even if the products had very specific sensory characteristics, including bitterness, astringency, and freshness, and the beer samples did not show any significant statistical difference, a beer with a higher Muscat Hamburg content was more desirable. Also, a higher phenolic content was observed in the sample produced with Muscat Hamburg. (Veljovic, 2016).

Veljovic et al. (2010) studied the possibility of producing and examining a beverage by wort fermentation enriched with grape must. They took must from two different varieties of grapes and added it to brewer's wort. The fermentation was carried out using a traditional method for lager beer production, with the entire process taking 30 days. Following the fermentation process, sensory analysis of the final product was performed, and the total polyphenol content was determined. These results suggested that it is possible to produce a pleasant beverage with some sensory properties similar to conventional beer. In addition to acceptable sensory properties, this drink was characterized by a higher alcohol (7–7.5% v/v) and polyphenol content.

A beer brewed from wort and the must of three grape varieties: Prokupac, Cabernet Sauvignon, and Pinot noir. *Saccharomyces cerevisiae* and *S. pastorianus* were used for the fermentation of beer, and it was observed that *S. pastorianus* showed more efficiency in wort metabolizing than *S. cerevisiae*. Beers containing grape must have seven-fold more phenolic compounds than the control beer. It was observed that beers having 20% (w/w) grape must have better sensory properties. And the consumption of these beers also acted favorably on heart rate and blood pressure, helping keep them normal (Rosul et al., 2019).

Cukalovic et al. (2010) evaluated the possible use of Ganoderma extract for the production of beer with enhanced biologically active ingredients and acceptable sensory properties. *Ganoderma lucidum* is unique among all cultivated mushrooms due to its medicinal and nutritional value. It was observed that its bioactive components and pharmacological functioning make it possible to use as a raw material for brewing a beer with improved functional properties. Ganoderma extract was produced, its main bioactive substance content was determined, and sensory evaluation of the final products enriched with it was performed. Consumers carried out the acceptance test. The sensory results indicated that both male and female tasters evaluated the enriched beer as similar to or better than the control beer. Male tasters showed great affinity for sensory properties like body, liveliness, and taste, whereas female tasters evaluated both beers quite similarly. Hence, beer with Ganoderma compared to a control beer differs statistically significantly only in its body.

Beer is a fermented beverage that, according to Jahn et al. (2020), can have antioxidants that contribute to the product's oxidative stability and nutraceutical qualities. They made a single malt pale ale and infused it with aronia berries under various process circumstances by introducing the antioxidant-rich fruits at different phases of the brewing process. The end product was a single malt pale ale with an aronia berry flavor. Aronia berries have a strong sour and astringent flavor, which limits their use in culinary applications because of their high antioxidant content. The polyphenol content as well as the antioxidant potential and color were assessed. There was a strong link between the amount of aronia that was added and the product's overall antioxidant capacity. Increased amounts of added aronia led to an increase in both the polyphenol content and the EBC color rating, but there was no discernible impact on the pH of the final product. During fermentation, a favorable effect on sugar utilization was demonstrated by an increase in the attenuation that was caused by an increase in the amount of aronia. The addition of aronia after the boil produced the best results in terms of coloration and antioxidative capacity, whereas the addition of aronia before the boil produced results that were comparable in terms of antioxidative capacity but had a lower EBC rating. When considered as a whole, the process of infusing pale ale with aronia berries has the potential to raise the beer's EBC rating, as well as its polyphenol content and antioxidative capacity.

There has been a boost in the consumption of craft beers due to the increase in craft breweries. But these beers face a drawback: with ageing, their flavors change. Compounds that overcome this downside can be used as an alternative. Piva et al. (2021) brewed pilsner beers with an increased shelf life using leaves of *Ocimum selloi*. These leaves are known for their antioxidant properties. Beers were brewed by adding in natura leaves or aqueous extract from the leaves of *Ocimum selloi*, and these beers were analyzed for volatiles and total phenolic compounds content, pH, color, and antioxidant activity. An increase in volatile content, improvement in the shelf life, and increase in the antioxidant potential of the beers was observed when the aqueous extract at 0.1% (m/v) was added after completion of the fermentation step.

Ulloa et al. (2017) added ethanolic extract of propolis to beer, using different concentrations (0.05, 0.15, and 0.25 g/l). The total phenolic content, total flavonoid content, and antioxidant activity of the beer samples were analyzed. The addition of extract of propolis to beer led to an increase in the total phenolic content with values of 4.5%, 16.7%, and 26.7% above a control. An increase in total flavonoid content was also observed (16.0%, 49.7%, and 59.2% above the control). A linear increase in antioxidant activity was observed with extract addition. No significant changes were observed in the physicochemical properties of golden ale beer with or without extract of propolis.

Dordevic et al. (2015) conducted research in which they added various plant extracts to beer. The results showed that beer containing lemon balm extract had the best sensory properties, while beer containing thyme extract was the most functional, in terms of the total amount of phenols and antioxidant activity it contained.

Scientific evidence indicates a cancer-preventive potential in selected hop-derived beer constituents, such as prenylflavonoids (xanthohumol and isoxanthohumol) and hops' bitter acids. Chemopreventive activities observed with these compounds were reported to be relevant in inhibiting carcinogenesis at the initiation, promotion, and progression phases. Therefore, all these studies corroborate the idea that beer may be a suitable alternative for consumers interested in the health benefits displayed by phenolic compounds and antioxidant activity.

Since several studies indicate that reactive oxygen species (ROS) and, consequently, oxidative stress are closely associated with a diverse assortment of diseases, and beers are able to increase antioxidant capacity in humans, the evaluation of such products is essential in order to provide information about their possible health benefits (Granato et al., 2011).

The use of by-products in the food industry can be an interesting alternative in the brewing of beer. Not only will this add economic value to wasted raw materials, but it also will reduce costs and environmental contamination problems while incorporating flavor and aroma into the beer (Helkar et al., 2016).

Gasiński et al. (2022) brewed beer with the addition of white grape pomace (the main by-product of white wine production), which possesses a high concentration of nutrients and bioactive substances. They added grape pomace in two different concentrations (10% w/w and 20% w/w) with two different pretreatments (pasteurized and unpasteurized) to the beer after primary fermentation and analyzed the use of the most abundant waste from the white wine industry to modify the volatile and phenolic content of the beer. The addition of white grape pomace led to an increase in the concentration of the phenolic compounds in beer (from 321.584 mg gallic acid equivalent (GAE)/L to 501.459 mg GAE/L). The antioxidant activity of the beers with grape pomace were tested using the ABTS, DPPH, and FRAP assays, and there was a significant increase observed. A change in the composition of the volatiles of beers upon grape pomace addition was observed. It was observed that the most significant difference was in the concentration of acetaldehyde; beers with grape pomace added had between four and seven times lower acetaldehyde content (17.425–31.425 mg/L) than the control sample (134.050 mg/L).

The antioxidant activity and phenolic content of beer depend on the quantity and quality of ingredients and on the method of brewing. Phenolic components also play a role in the color, taste, and stability of beer (Callemien et al., 2005). Beers rich in phenolic components are of higher quality have more stability in terms of flavor and foam, and have a longer shelf life.

Koren et al. (2017) studied 40 Hungarian retail beers for folic acid content, antioxidant profile, and physicochemical parameters. They reported the lowest physicochemical parameters, folic acid content, and antioxidant activity in alcohol-free beers. They observed that beers aged with sour cherries had the highest folic acid content. Dark beers and beers that were aged with sour cherries showed the highest antioxidant activity, probably due to their high extract content, the fruits components that were responsible for antioxidant activity, and special malts. Their results highlighted a possible way to achieve adequate folic acid and relevant antioxidant intake without excessive alcohol and energy consumption by choosing appropriate beer types.

Nishant et al., conducted a doctoral study on the effects of incorporating different fruits into the wort, and surprisingly positive results were found in the final product. The lab samples were compared beers with already available on the market.

Beer is a very good source of antioxidants, and the composition of its antioxidants depends not only on the raw materials but also on the technology used to produce it (Jurková et al., 2012). Fruit juices and other beverages have high concentrations of natural antioxidants, including polyphenols (Ramadan-Hassanien, 2008). The polyphenol compounds of beer are mainly derived from malt (75%) and hops (25%) and influence some traits in beer like its color, taste, and bitterness (Nizet et al., 2013).

In this study, all the brewed beers were analyzed for total polyphenol content by the Folin-Ciocalteu method and for antioxidant activity by the ABTS, FRAP, and DPPH methods. The results are presented in Table 7.1.

TABLE 7.1
Polyphenol Content and Antioxidant Activity

Beer	Total Polyphenols (mg GAE/L)	ABTS (mmol TE/L)	FRAP (mmol TE/L)	DPPH (mmol TE/L)
LB	212.8 ± 11.3[a]	1.32 ± 0.9[a]	0.96 ± 3.1[a]	1.52 ± 4.1[a]
CL	337.6 ± 20.9[b]	1.85 ± 2.3[b]	1.89 ± 1.6[b]	2.37 ± 3.9[c]
WB	236.1 ± 13.1[a]	1.21 ± 1.1[a]	1.03 ± 2.9[a]	2.01 ± 1.9[b]
CWB	253.3 ± 23.7[a]	1.36 ± 2.3[a]	1.15 ± 3.3[a]	2.26 ± 2.3[c]
AB	382.2 ± 12.5[c]	2.61 ± 0.5[c]	1.97 ± 1.3[b]	2.87 ± 5.3[c]
DB	409.3 ± 17.6[c]	1.96 ± 1.5[b]	2.30 ± 2.1[c]	2.92 ± 1.4[d]
BBB	335.8 ± 9.3[b]	1.72 ± 0.7[b]	1.87 ± 0.9[b]	2.06 ± 3.8[c]
KB	385.6 ± 15.6[c]	2.09 ± 2.6[b]	2.21 ± 2.3[c]	2.39 ± 5.9[c]

*All the results were statistically analyzed.

However, hops were also a source of antioxidant compounds (e.g., polyphenols) (Krofta et al., 2008), but we have used the same hops in the same quantity in all beers.

As shown in Table 7.1, the total polyphenols in all the analyzed beers were in the range of 212.8–409.3 mg GAE/L; the lowest for lager beer and dark beer has highest among all beer samples. It was observed that the addition of fruits and dark malts led to an increase in total polyphenols as well as antioxidant activity.

Similar results were observed by Pereira et al. (2020). An increase in polyphenol content in beers with cashew peduncle was observed; this increased with an increase in the concentration of cashew peduncle in the beer. It was observed that beers with 10% cashew peduncle had higher polyphenol content than those with 5%. This is due to the presence of considerable amounts of phenolic compounds in the cashew peduncle. However, it was observed that beers with 0.6% orange peel did not show any significant difference from the control. A combination of both cashew peduncle and orange peel bioactive compounds acted synergistically and had a greater effect on antioxidant activity, as it was observed that beers with 5% cashew peduncle and 0.6% orange peel had higher antioxidant activity than the control.

Nardini and Garaguso (2020) analyzed the polyphenol content and antioxidant activity of various fruit beers and observed total polyphenol content in the range of 399–767 mg/L in the fruit beers, which was much higher than that of conventional beers, which are in the range 321–482 mg/L beer. It was observed that cherry beers had the highest polyphenol content, followed by orange, then grape, plum, raspberry, peach, apricot, and apple beers.

Results obtained in our study were in agreement with the results reported by Ducruet et al. (2017), who observed a higher concentration of phenolic compounds in beers brewed with goji berries than in the control beer. The total phenolic content was in the range of 335 mg GAE/L for the standard amber ale, which is quite similar to our results, to 623 mg GAE/L for the beer with goji berries added at the beginning of the wort boiling. There was no significant difference found between beers using

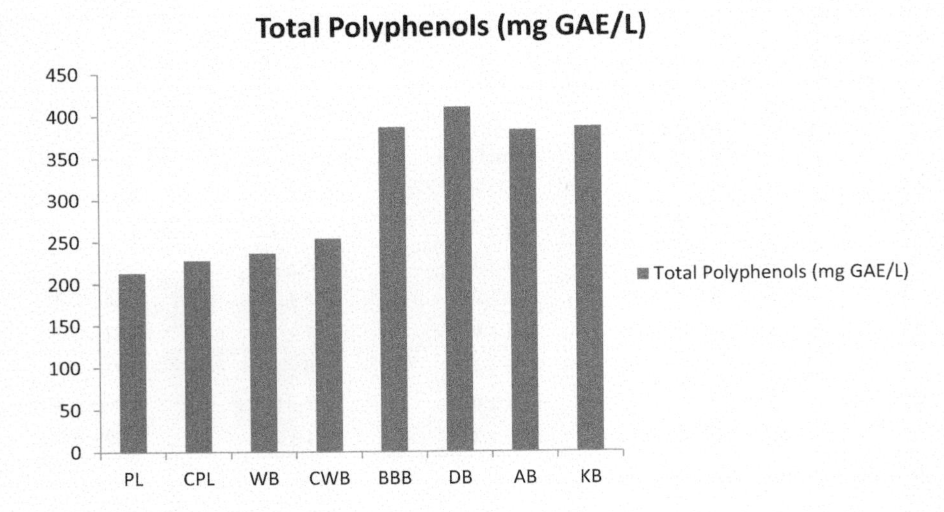

FIGURE 7.1 Total Polyphenol Content of All Beers

ground and whole goji berries. Also, there were no significant differences in the total phenolic content of beers with goji berries added at the first stage of fermentation and beers with goji berries added at the bottling line.

The antioxidant capacity of the beer samples was analyzed by ABTS and oxygen radical absorbance capacity (ORAC) assays. It was observed that TEAC values for beer samples ranged from 2.26 to 3.82 mmol/L, whereas ORAC was from 8.87 to 8.87 to 16.84 mmol/L. It was also reported that the addition of 50 g/L of goji berries resulted in a significant increase in the antioxidant capacity of the beer. But the addition of 11 g/L of crushed goji berries just before bottling did not show any significant change in the antioxidant capacity (Ducruet et al., 2017).

Socha et al. (2017) analyzed hydrolyzed and non-hydrolyzed samples of dark beers for antioxidant activity by using both ABTS and DPPH assays. It was reported that the antioxidant activity of hydrolyzed beer samples was much greater than that of the non-hydrolyzed ones. This is due to alkaline hydrolysis; phenolic compounds of beer decompose to their free forms (i.e., phenolic acids and aglycone of flavonoids). It was also observed that the antioxidant activity of hydrolyzed and non-hydrolyzed samples of different dark beers (brand-wise) have great variation. This is because of the use of different raw materials (e.g., barley and hops, etc.), as well as the use of different brewing processes in those beer samples.

Koren et al. (2017) reported the highest antioxidant activity in dark beers and beers aged with sour cherry (ranging from 427.91 to 1033.66 mg/L GAE) and the lowest in alcohol-free beers and beer-based mixed drinks. Similar results were observed by Granato et al. (2011); dark beers exhibited higher antioxidant activity (280–525 mg/L GAE) than pale beers (119–200 mg/L GAE). This difference in antioxidant activity of beers was due to the various special malts, like crystal, black or caramel, used in their production. These special malts are malted by giving specific time and

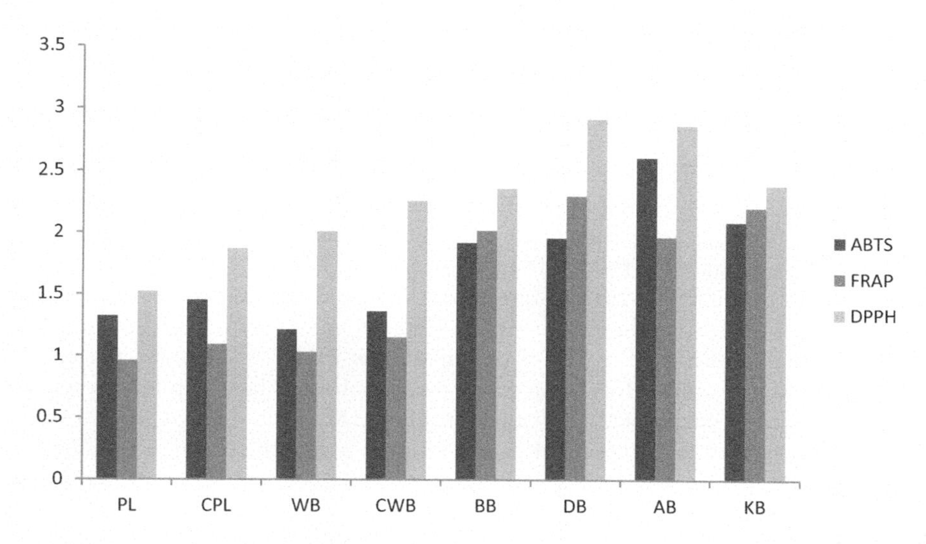

FIGURE 7.2 Antioxidant Activity of All Beers (in mmol TE/L)

temperature profiles at the time of the kilning and roasting processes, due to which different compounds are generated via the Maillard reaction, which has antioxidant activity (Tubaro, 2009).

Beers with sour cherry exhibited higher antioxidant activity mostly due to the antioxidant compounds (anthocyanins) present in fruits. Usually, alcohol-free and low-alcohol beers are brewed using special malts that have low extract content and are lightly hopped. This might be why they exhibited the lowest antioxidant activity of these beers (Koren et al., 2017). But the product containing blackcurrant juice showed the highest antioxidant activity among alcohol-free beers. This is owing to the high antioxidant activity of blackcurrant juice, which is high in phenolic compounds and ascorbic acid, which have antioxidant activity (Mattila et al., 2011).

Also, Gasinski et al. (2020) analyzed and observed the highest total polyphenol content in beers with mango and reported the highest antioxidant activity in beers with mango juice (44% higher than the control) among all tested samples. It was also observed that that the addition of mango fruit in different forms leads to an increase in the polyphenol content of beer.

Kawa-Rygielska et al. (2019) observed higher polyphenols concentration in worts with Cornelian cherry juice than in the control. The highest was in the wort with the juice of red fruits, the wort with yellow fruits was slightly lower, followed by wort with coral fruits; the lowest was in the control beer.

But Martínez et al. (2017) observed that the addition of persimmon fruits during brewing decreases the total polyphenol concentration in the finished product and that reduction gradually increases with the addition of more fruits. This is due to the persimmon fruits not having phenolic compounds.

Antioxidant activity analyzed using both ABTS and FRAP methods was observed higher in fruit beers, ranging from 1.62 to 3.53 mM Trolox/L beer for the ABTS assay and from 3.08 to 9.76 mM Fe_2SO_4/L beer for the FRAP assay. The highest antioxidant activity was observed with the ABTS assay in cherry beers, followed by grape, raspberry, plum, orange, peach, apricot, and apple beers. A similar pattern of results was observed in the FRAP assay: conventional beers had lower antioxidant activity than that of fruit beers, in the ranges of 1.29–2.03 mM Trolox/L beer for the ABTS assay and 2.80–4.39 mM Fe_2SO_4/L beer for the FRAP assay.

Numerous studies have been done on the total phenolic content and antioxidant capacities of commercial beers (Granato et al., 2011; Pai et al., 2015; Tafulo et al., 2010; Zhao et al., 2010, 2013). Many results showed large differences between beer types, but also within one beer type. Piazzon et al. (2010) analyzed antioxidant activities in different types of beer using the FRAP assay and reported an increasing activity in the following order: dealcoholized < lager < pilsner < wheat < ale < abbey < bock beer. The values in the TEAC assay ranged from 0.16 to 2.23 mmol/L TE for Chinese and exported lager beer (Zhao et al., 2010, 2013). Values of 0.64–1.08 and 14.2–25.7 mmol/L for ABTS and ORAC, respectively, were reported for Belgian ale (Tafulo et al., 2010).

In general, ale has a much higher antioxidant capacity than lager (Granato et al., 2011). The ORAC value obtained in the present study for standard amber ale beer (control beer F) was almost as high as that reported for the most active Brazilian ale, ORAC values 0.7–10.5 mmol/L (Granato et al., 2011).

Similarly, large differences in total phenolic content were found in the literature. The lowest values were noted for Chinese lager: i.e., 84.64–267.27 mg GAE/L (Zhao et al., 2013). The values closer to those obtained in this study were reported for Indian ale (160–620 mg GAE/L) (Pai et al., 2015) and Brazilian ale (117–526 mg GAE/L) (Granato et al., 2011).

Piazzon et al. (2010) analyzed five different brands of each of the seven beer types (dealcoholized, lager, pilsner, wheat, ale, abbey, and bock). They reported that the total polyphenol content differed significantly, depending on the beer type, ranging from 366 GAE mg/L for dealcoholized beers to 875 GAE mg/L for bock beers. The polyphenol content was significantly higher in abbey and ale beers than in dealcoholized beers. They reported that the antioxidant activity of the beers, measured by the FRAP assay, was similar to the polyphenol content, the ferric ion reducing antioxidant activity of beers also showed significant differences depending on beer type, ranging from 1,525 µmol of $Fe2^{+/L}$ for dealcoholized beers to 4,663 µmol of $Fe2^{+/L}$ for bock beers. The measured antioxidant activity in bock beers was highest, followed by abbey beers and ale.

Gasior et al. (2020) reported that the polyphenol content in worts with 10% of additive was 176.02–397.03 mg GAE/L, ferric reducing antioxidant power (FRAP) 1.32–2.07 mmol TE/L, and capacity to reduce radicals generated from 2,20-Azino-bis (3-ethylbenzothiazoline-6-sulfonic acid) diammonium salt (ABTS) 1.46–2.70 mmol TE/L.

7.2 PHENOLIC PROFILE ANALYSES

Polyphenols are natural antioxidants and greatly affect the quality of beer. The antioxidant properties of malt and beer are usually associated with phenolic compounds

(Rivero et al., 2005). In fact, phenolic acids have been reported as strong antioxidants due to their ability to donate hydrogen and electrons and also due to the formation of stable radical intermediates, which prevent oxidation of other compounds (Maillard & Berset, 1995; Subba Rao & Muralikrishna, 2002). Still, compounds with a flavonoid structure have generally shown higher antioxidant activity than non-flavonoid compounds (Zhao et al., 2010), mainly determined by their hydroxyl groups (Fukumoto & Mazza, 2000; Qingming et al., 2010).

So beer samples were analyzed to determine the profile of phenolic acids and flavonoids by HPLC. The hydroxycinnamic acid derivatives vanillic, caffeic, and p-coumaric; the hydroxybenzoic acid derivative syringic; and the flavonoids catechin and quercetin were measured. These phenolic acids were chosen because they presented higher concentrations in several studies on beers (Nardini & Garaguso, 2020; Zhang et al., 2013; Zhao et al., 2010; Piazzon et al., 2010; Szwajgier, 2009).

First, if we compare analyzed polyphenols, gallic acid was observed in the highest range of 22.8–160 mg/L, followed by caffeic (2.0–5.10 mg/L), vanillic (2.0–12.70 mg/L), p-coumaric (1.0–2.40 mg/L), and syringic (1.0–2.26 mg/L). Among flavonoids, catechin was observed in a range of 1.1–11.96 mg/L, and quercetin was in the range of 0–6 mg/L.

The control beer sample showed the lowest content of gallic acid, syringic, and p-coumaric acids compared to both dark and fruit beers. These results are in agreement with those reported in previous studies (Nardini & Ghiselli, 2004; Piazzon et al., 2010).

Nardini and Garaguso (2020) also observed that total ferulic acid was by far the most abundant phenolic acid in conventional beers, regardless of the beer style, ranging from 9.97 to 22.6 mg/L, followed by caffeic acid (1.86–6.38 mg/L), vanillic acid (1.47–5.45 mg/L), sinapic acid (2.44–4.87 mg/L) and p-coumaric acid (0.92–3.10 mg/L) while syringic acid exhibited the lowest concentration (0.49–0.89 mg/L). It was reported that lager beers have lower caffeic, syringic, and p-coumaric acids than lambic- and ale-style beers. Phenolic acids in beers are mainly in conjugated form. Also, it was observed that the total amount of each phenolic acid after alkaline

TABLE 7.2
Phenolic Profile of Beers

Phenolic Compounds (mg/L)								
	LB	CL	WB	CWB	AB	DB	BBB	KB
Vanillic	1.96	1.3	1.1	1.8	5.56	2	2.82	2.70
Gallic Acid	24.4	22.8	47	36	134.63	160	42	83
Syringic	1.05	1.0	1.0	1.0	1.81	2	2.07	1.26
Caffeic	2.63	3.4	2	3	4.05	18	2.74	5.10
P-coumaric	1.15	0.9	1.12	3	3.14	2.87	1.26	1.40
Flavonoids (mg/L)								
Catechin	1.42	1.1	3	7	11.96	6	2.23	6.75
Quercetin	0.72	0.1	6	6	3.83	1	0.85	2.46

hydrolysis was higher than the respective free form. The flavonoids like catechin, rutin, myricetin, and quercetin and the stilbene derivative resveratrol were undetectable in all conventional no-fruit beers, regardless of the beer style.

The content of every single phenolic acid was different among all the fruit types, and the total phenolic acids obtained after alkaline hydrolysis were in the range of 26.51–145.8 mg/L beer, with cherry, plum, grape, and orange beers exhibiting the highest values.

Total caffeic acid content ranged from 2.77 to 89.9 mg/L beer and considerably higher in most of the fruit beers, particularly plum, cherry, apricot, peach, and grape, while the values measured in orange, apple, and raspberry beers were close to those found in conventional beers (range 1.86–6.38 mg/L).

Total p-coumaric content ranged from 1.25 to 62.4 mg/L beer, and it was particularly high in cherry beers. followed by plum, grape, raspberry, and orange beers, when compared to the content of conventional beers.

The total ferulic acid (9.23–27.87 mg/L) and vanillic acid (2.68–6.98 mg/L) content of fruit beers (Table 7.2) were quite close to those of the conventional group (9.97–22.6 mg/L and 1.47–5.45 mg/L for ferulic and sinapic acids, respectively).

The total syringic acid content of fruit beers (0.50–2.46 mg/L beer) was higher than that of conventional beers (0.49–0.89 mg/L) (Table 7.1), with grape beer showing the highest value (2.46 mg/L beer) (Table 7.2).

For each phenolic acid, the total amount measured after alkaline hydrolysis is higher than the content of the respective free form, indicating that phenolic acids are mainly present as conjugated forms in fruit beers also.

Unlike conventional beers, both chlorogenic and neo-chlorogenic acids were present in most fruit beers (0.81–12.71 mg/L and 0.79–60.3 mg/L for chlorogenic and neo-chlorogenic acids, respectively). The highest level of chlorogenic acid was measured in apricot beer (12.71 mg/L), followed by cherry and plum beers. Plum beer exhibited the highest value of neo-chlorogenic acid content (60.3 mg/L), followed by cherry and apricot beers.

The flavonoids catechin and quercetin were present in all fruit beers. Catechin levels ranged from 1.00 to 20.4 mg/L beer, with the highest value measured in cherry beer, followed by orange, apricot, grape, plum, raspberry, peach, and apple beers. Quercetin content was in the range 0.30–7.10 mg/L, with the highest values measured in cherry beers, followed by apricot, raspberry (RASP1), grape, plum, apple, and peach beers. The myricetin content of fruit beers varied in the range 0.76–5.31 mg/L beer, with the highest value measured in plum beer, while only trace amounts were detected in grape, apple, and raspberry beers. Under our experimental conditions, the flavonoid rutin was undetectable or present only in trace amounts in most of the fruit beers, except apple and orange beers, which exhibited concentrations of 0.56 and 1.49 mg/L beer, respectively. With respect to the stilbene derivative resveratrol, the highest level was measured in grape beer (2.24 mg/L), followed by peach, apple, raspberry, cherry, and apricot beers. Under our experimental conditions, resveratrol was undetectable in orange and plum beers.

Piazzon et al. (2010) analyzed a subset of 21 beers (three different brands for each of the seven beer types) for the content of both free and total phenolic acids using

HPLC-ECD and reported that the most abundant phenolic acid in beers was ferulic acid, followed by vanillic, caffeic, and p-coumaric. Ferulic, caffeic, and syringic acids are present in beers mainly as bound forms, whereas p-coumaric is generally present equally in bound and free forms. They reported that the phenolic acid content was significantly different in beers samples depending on type, dealcoholized beers having lowest and bock beer the highest levels among all the samples. It was reported that catechin was in 5 beers out of 21 beers in the range of 0.1–2.6 mg/L.

In this study, it was observed that the addition of fruit that is rich in polyphenols and antioxidant activity led to an increase in the same in the finished product as well.

Nardini and Garaguso (2020) studied different types of beers; ale showed the highest total polyphenol content and antioxidant activity while lager exhibited the lowest. Lambic beers were also higher in polyphenol content than the lager style while antioxidant activity was less than in other beers. Fruit beers (mostly) showed the highest antioxidant activity, total polyphenol and flavonoid content among the beers. The phenolic profile obtained by HPLC showed that phenolic acids are usually higher in fruit beers than in other non-fruit beers, except for ferulic acid, which is present in almost similar concentration in non-fruit and fruit beers.

Vinson et al. (2003) showed that polyphenols present in both lager and dark beer (225 mL per day) significantly inhibited atherosclerosis, decreased both total cholesterol and triglycerides in serum, acted as in vivo antioxidant by decreasing the oxidizability of low-density lipoprotein cholesterol, and decreased atherosclerosis compared to the 0.4% alcohol control in cholesterol-fed hamsters. Lager beer also inhibited atherosclerosis at a human-equivalent dose in this hamster model of atherosclerosis. It was shown that consumption of 500 mL of 4.5% ethanol Italian lager beer in the morning increases antioxidant capacity one hour after consumption and increases plasma phenolic acid levels (caffeic, sinapic, syringic, and vanillic acids) for up to two hours after consumption, thus increasing antioxidant activity in the body. The increase in antioxidant capacity is not caused by ethanol alone or by dealcoholized beer, showing there is a synergism between its components whereby ethanol increases absorption of phenolic acids. Beer was found to affect plasma lipid profiles and plasma antioxidant capacity positively and to increase bile excretion in rats fed cholesterol-containing diets.

Nardini and Garaguso (2020) found that caffeic acid content was high in most of the fruit beers, so it might be possible that it contributes to antioxidant activity of fruit beers. Plum and cherry beers showed the highest caffeic acid content. In the case of flavonoids, only catechin and quercetin were observed in all fruit beer samples and myricetin in 7 out of 10 fruit beers, while rutin is present in orange and apple beers.

Flavonoids also act as free radical scavengers and strong antioxidants (Kumar & Pandey, 2013). So the increase in flavonoids observed in most of the fruit beers led to the higher antioxidant activity.

Cherry beers exhibited the highest phenolic content among fruit beers. In the case of orange beer, the amount of fruit used was less (5 g orange peels/L beer) than in other fruit beers, but it showed higher antioxidant activity, total polyphenols, and flavonoid content.

Grape beer showed the highest antioxidant activity and total flavonoid content after cherry beers. Moreover, all values measured in grape beer were markedly higher than those measured in the conventional ales that were used by the manufacturer for grape beer production, outlining the major contribution of fruit to the nutritional quality of beer.

Gasinski et al. (2020) brewed and studied beer having mango fruit (*Mangifera indica*). The effect of mango addition on the volatile composition of beer was also observed. They used mango fruit in beer in five different forms and observed which improved beer aroma. They reported that beer without mango had the lowest volatile compounds content (1787.84 μg/100 mL), whereas beer prepared with mango pulp had the highest concentration of volatile components from mango (2112.15 μg/100 mL). Mango addition leads to an increase in the concentration of α-pinene, β-myrcene, terpinolene, α-terpineol, cis-β-ocimene, caryophyllene, and humulene in the final beer. They also reported that beers with mango added had a polyphenol content 44% higher than the control beer and also a higher antioxidant activity than the control.

Raspberry beers also showed higher antioxidant activity and total polyphenols than non-fruit beers. The two raspberry beers were brewed with different quantities of fruit: 300 g raspberries/l beer in first one and 100 g raspberries/l beer in second.

Kawa-Rygielska et al. (2019) studied the use of Cornelian cherry juices in brewing technology. They analyzed the basic physicochemical properties, the concentration of polyphenols and iridoids, and the antioxidative activity of brewed beer. The concentration of total polyphenols (F-C) in Cornelian cherry beer ranged from 398.1 to 688.7 mg GAE/L beer. The antioxidative activity measured with the FRAP and DPPH assays was the highest in the beer with the addition of juice from the red-fruit cultivar. Among all the identified iridoids, loganic acid was the predominating one, and its highest concentration, 184.6 mg LA/L beer, was observed in the beer with juice made of the coral-fruit cultivar. These identified polyphenols included anthocyanins and flavonol derivatives. The novelty of their study was brewing beers containing compounds from the group of iridoids.

Adadi et al. (2017) brewed a non-traditional beer supplemented with sea buckthorns. After one month of primary fermentation, they added sea buckthorns that were sanitized and crashed before adding. They analyzed the physicochemical properties, microbial load, and sensory evaluation of the fruit beer and observed that there was a significant influence on the physicochemical properties of beer upon the addition of sea buckthorns. They identified 32 volatile compounds. Even during sensory analysis, it was preferred by the panelists. It also showed higher DPPH radical scavenging activity as compared than other types.

According to Nardini and Garaguso (2020), fruit addition during the fermentation step led to considerable improvement in nutritional quality of beer, especially the content of bioactive compounds and antioxidant activity. This increase is beneficial for beer consumers.

Various studies confirm that there is quick absorption of the phenolic acids present in beer by the human body, and they are extensively metabolized to glucuronide and sulfate derivatives (Bourne et al., 2000; Nardini et al., 2006). Flavonoids, the most abundant polyphenol (antioxidant) present in human diets, are absorbed in humans and then circulate in plasma and are excreted in urine (Scalbert & Williamson,

2000). It has been reported that flavonoids exhibit antioxidant activity, free radical–scavenging capacity, and coronary heart disease prevention (Kumar & Pandey, 2013; Williamson & Manach, 2005). Mild to moderate alcohol consumption is associated with beneficial effects on the cardiovascular system (Arranz et al., 2012; Kaplan et al., 2000).

Nardini and Garaguso (2020) concluded that beer contributes to the overall dietary intake of antioxidants, and beer having fruits increases this contribution.

Innovation is the key driver in all industries. There is a constant increase in demand for new products in the market: a new flavor, more attractive packaging, improved quality, more health benefits. Nowadays, due to the increase in people aspiring to live a healthy lifestyle, there is a regular demand for healthy food, and functional food is becoming a very important concept.

The addition of various herbs (hops, sweet gale, etc.) to beer dates back to the Middle Ages when people wanted to obtain a new beer. The flavor of beer becomes more pleasant when it is mixed with some aromatic herbs (Djordjevic et al., 2016).

The addition of herbs with antioxidative properties to beers also increases their antioxidant capacity. Belščak-Cvitanović et al. (2017) encapsulated green tea extracts using electrostatic extrusion and dry green tea extracts using spray drying. The control beer samples were lemon Radler and pilsner beer. A slight increase was reported in total phenolic content in all the beers with extracts. The best sensory qualities among the samples was in Radler beer with green tea as it was the least bitter and had a stronger, pleasant herbal note in taste.

7.3 REFERENCES

Adadi, P., Kovaleva, E. G., Glukhareva, T. V., Shatunova, S. A., & Petrov, A. S. (2017). Production and analysis of non-traditional beer supplemented with sea buckthorn. *Agronomy Research*, *15*(5), 1831–1845.

Arranz, S., Chiva-Blanch, G., Valderas-Martínez, P., Medina-Remón, A., Lamuela-Raventós, R. M., & Estruch, R. (2012). Wine, beer, alcohol and polyphenols on cardiovascular disease and cancer. *Nutrients*, *4*(7), 759–781.

Belščak-Cvitanović, A., Nedović, V., Salević, A., Despotović, S., Komes, D., Nikšić, M., Bugarski, B., & Leskošek-Čukalović, I. (2017). Modification of functional quality of beer by using microencapsulated green tea (Camellia sinensis L.) and Ganoderma mushroom (Ganoderma lucidum L.) bioactive compounds. *Chemical Industry & Chemical Engineering Quarterly*, *23*(4), 457–471.

Bourne, L., Paganga, G., Baxter, D., Hughes, P., & Rice-Evans, C. (2000). Absorption of ferulic acid from low-alcohol beer. *Free Radical Research*, *32*(3), 273–280.

Callemien, D., Jerkovic, V., Rozenberg, R., & Collin, S. (2005). Hop as an interesting source of resveratrol for brewers: Optimization of the extraction and quantitative study by liquid chromatography/atmospheric pressure chemical ionization tandem mass spectrometry. *Journal of Agricultural and Food Chemistry*, *53*(2), 424–429.

Cukalovic, I. L., Despotovic, S., Lakic, N., Niksic, M., Nedovic, V., & Tesevic, V. (2010). Ganoderma lucidum—medical mushroom as a raw material for beer with enhanced functional properties. *Food Research International*, *43*(9), 2262–2269.

Djordjevic, S., Popović, D., Despotović, S., Veljović, M., Atanacković, M., Cvejić, J., Nedović, V., & Leskošek-Čukalović, I. (2016). Extracts of medicinal plants as functional beer additives. *Chemical Industry and Chemical Engineering Quarterly/CICEQ*, *22*(3), 301–308.

Dordevic, S., Popovic, D., Despotovic, S., Veljovic, M., & Atanackovic, M. (2015). Extracts of medicinal plants-as functional beer additives. *Chemical Industry and Chemical Engineering Quarterly*, 44–65.

Ducruet, J., Rébénaque, P., Diserens, S., Kosińska-Cagnazzo, A., Héritier, I., & Andlauer, W. (2017). Amber ale beer enriched with goji berries–The effect on bioactive compound content and sensorial properties. *Food Chemistry*, *226*, 109–118.

Fukumoto, L. R., & Mazza, G. (2000). Assessing antioxidant and prooxidant activities of phenolic compounds. *Journal of Agricultural and Food Chemistry*, *48*(8), 3597–3604.

Gasinski, A., Kawa-Rygielska, J., Szumny, A., Gąsior, J., & Głowacki, A. (2020). Assessment of volatiles and polyphenol content, physicochemical parameters and antioxidant activity in beers with dotted hawthorn (Crataegus punctata). *Foods*, *9*(6), 775.

Gasiński, A., Kawa-Rygielska, J., Mikulski, D., Kłosowski, G., & Głowacki, A. (2022). Application of white grape pomace in the brewing technology and its impact on the concentration of esters and alcohols, physicochemical parameteres and antioxidative properties of the beer. *Food Chemistry*, *367*, 130646.

Granato, D., Branco, G. F., Faria, J. D. A. F., & Cruz, A. G. (2011). Characterization of Brazilian lager and brown ale beers based on color, phenolic compounds, and antioxidant activity using chemometrics. *Journal of the Science of Food and Agriculture*, *91*(3), 563–571.

Habschied, K., Zivkovic, A., Krstanovic, V., & Mastanjevic, K. (2020). Functional beer—a review on possibilities. *Beverages*, *6*(3), 51.

Helkar, P. B., Sahoo, A. K., & Patil, N. J. (2016). Review: Food industry by-products used as a functional food ingredient. *International Journal of Waste Resources*, *6*(3), 1–6.

Jahn, A., Kim, J., & Bashir, K. M. I. (2020). Antioxidant content of aronia infused beer. *Fermentation*, *6*(3), 71.

Jurková, M., Horák, T., Hašková, D., Čulík, J., Čejka, P., & Kellner, V. (2012). Control of antioxidant beer activity by the mashing process. *Journal of the Institute of Brewing*, *118*(2), 230–235.

Kaplan, N. M., Palmer, B. F., & Denke, M. A. (2000). Nutritional and health benefits of beer. *American Journal of the Medical Sciences*, *320*(5), 320–326.

Kawa-Rygielska, J., Adamenko, K., Kucharska, A. Z., Prorok, P., & Piórecki, N. (2019). Physicochemical and antioxidative properties of Cornelian cherry beer. *Food Chemistry*, *281*, 147–153.

Koren, D., Orbán, C., Galló, N., Kun, S., Vecseri-Hegyes, B., & Kun-Farkas, G. (2017). Folic acid content and antioxidant activity of different types of beers available in Hungarian retail. *Journal of Food Science and Technology*, *54*(5), 1158–1167.

Krofta, K., Mikyška, A., & Hašková, D. (2008). Antioxidant characteristics of hops and hop products. *Journal of the Institute of Brewing*, *114*(2), 160–166.

Kumar, S., & Pandey, A. K. (2013). Chemistry and biological activities of flavonoids: An overview. *The Scientific World Journal, 2013*, 1–16.

Maillard, M. N., & Berset, C. (1995). Evolution of antioxidant activity during kilning: Role of insoluble bound phenolic acids of barley and malt. *Journal of Agricultural and Food Chemistry*, *43*(7), 1789–1793.

Martínez, A., Vegara, S., Herranz-López, M., Martí, N., Valero, M., Micol, V., & Saura, D. (2017). Kinetic changes of polyphenols, anthocyanins and antioxidant capacity in forced aged hibiscus ale beer. *Journal of the Institute of Brewing*, *123*(1), 58–65.

Mattila, P. H., Hellström, J., McDougall, G., Dobson, G., Pihlava, J. M., Tiirikka, T., Stewart, D., & Karjalainen, R. (2011). Polyphenol and vitamin C contents in European commercial blackcurrant juice products. *Food Chemistry*, *127*(3), 1216–1223.

Nardini, M., & Garaguso, I. (2020). Characterization of bioactive compounds and antioxidant activity of fruit beers. *Food Chemistry*, *305*, 125437.

Nardini, M., & Ghiselli, A. (2004). Determination of free and bound phenolic acids in beer. *Food Chemistry*, *84*(1), 137–143.

Nardini, M., Natella, F., Scaccini, C., & Ghiselli, A. (2006). Phenolic acids from beer are absorbed and extensively metabolized in humans. *The Journal of Nutritional Biochemistry*, *17*(1), 14–22.

Nizet, S., Gros, J., Peeters, F., Chaumont, S., Robiette, R., & Collin, S. (2013). First evidence of the production of odorant polyfunctional thiols by bottle refermentation. *Journal of the American Society of Brewing Chemists*, *71*(1), 15–22.

Pai, T. V., Sawant, S. Y., Ghatak, A. A., Chaturvedi, P. A., Gupte, A. M., & Desai, N. S. (2015). Characterization of Indian beers: Chemical composition and antioxidant potential. *Journal of Food Science and Technology*, *52*(3), 1414–1423.

Paiva, R. A., Mutz, Y. S., & Conte-Junior, C. A. (2021). A review on the obtaining of functional beers by addition of non-cereal adjuncts rich in antioxidant compounds. *Antioxidants*, *10*(9), 1332.

Pereira, I. M. C., Matos Neto, J. D., Figueiredo, R. W., Carvalho, J. D. G., Figueiredo, E. A. T. D., Menezes, N. V. S. D., & Gaban, S. V. F. (2020). Physicochemical characterization, antioxidant activity, and sensory analysis of beers brewed with cashew peduncle (Anacardium occidentale) and orange peel (Citrus sinensis). *Food Science and Technology*, *40*, 749–755.

Piazzon, A., Forte, M., & Nardini, M. (2010). Characterization of phenolics content and antioxidant activity of different beer types. *Journal of Agricultural and Food Chemistry*, *58*(19), 10677–10683.

Piva, R. C., Verdan, M. H., Mascarenhas Santos, M. D. S., Batistote, M., & Cardoso, C. A. L. (2021). Manufacturing and characterization of craft beers with leaves from Ocimum selloi Benth. *Journal of Food Science and Technology*, *58*(11), 4403–4410.

Qingming, Y., Xianhui, P., Weibao, K., Hong, Y., Yidan, S., Li, Z., Yanan, Z., Yuling, Y., Lan, D., & Guoan, L. (2010). Antioxidant activities of malt extract from barley (Hordeum vulgare L.) toward various oxidative stress in vitro and in vivo. *Food Chemistry*, *118*(1), 84–89.

Ramadan-Hassanien, M. F. (2008). Total antioxidant potential of juices, beverages and hot drinks consumed in Egypt screened by DPPH in vitro assay. *Grasas y Aceites*, *59*(3), 254–259.

Rivero, D., Pérez-Magariño, S., González-Sanjosé, M. L., Valls-Belles, V., Codoñer, P., & Muñiz, P. (2005). Inhibition of induced DNA oxidative damage by beers: Correlation with the content of polyphenols and melanoidins. *Journal of Agricultural and Food Chemistry*, *53*(9), 3637–3642.

Rosul, M. Đ., Mandić, A. I., Mišan, A. Č., Đerić, N. R., & Pejin, J. D. (2019). Review of trends in formulation of functional beer. *Food and Feed Research*, *46*(1), 23–35.

Scalbert, A., & Williamson, G. (2000). Dietary intake and bioavailability of polyphenols. *The Journal of Nutrition*, *130*(8), 2073S–2085S.

Socha, R., Pająk, P., Fortuna, T., & Buksa, K. (2017). Antioxidant activity and the most abundant phenolics in commercial dark beers. *International Journal of Food Properties*, *20*(sup1), S595–S609.

Subba Rao, M. V. S. S. T., & Muralikrishna, G. (2002). Evaluation of the antioxidant properties of free and bound phenolic acids from native and malted finger millet (Ragi, Eleusine coracana Indaf-15). *Journal of Agricultural and Food Chemistry*, *50*(4), 889–892.

Szwajgier, D. (2009). Content of individual phenolic acids in worts and beers and their possible contribution to the antiradical activity of beer. *Journal of the Institute of Brewing*, *115*(3), 243–252.

Tafulo, P. A. R., Queirós, R. B., Delerue-Matos, C. M., & Sales, M. G. F. (2010). Control and comparison of the antioxidant capacity of beers. *Food Research International*, *43*(6), 1702–1709.

Tubaro, F. (2009). Antioxidant activity of beer's Maillard reaction products: Features and health aspects. In *Beer in health and disease prevention* (pp. 449–457). Academic Press.

Ulloa, P. A., Vidal, J., Ávila, M. I., Labbe, M., Cohen, S., & Salazar, F. N. (2017). Effect of the addition of propolis extract on bioactive compounds and antioxidant activity of craft beer. *Journal of Chemistry*, *2017*, 7. https://doi.org/10.1155/2017/6716053.

Veljovic, M. (2016). *Chemical, functional and sensory properties of beer enriched with biologically active compounds of grape* [Doctoral dissertation, Faculty of Agriculture, University of Belgrade].

Veljovic, M., Djordjevic, R., Leskosek-Cukalovic, I., Lakic, N., Despotovic, S., Pecic, S., & Nedovic, V. (2010). The possibility of producing a special type of beer made from wort with the addition of grape must. *Journal of the Institute of Brewing*, *116*(4), 440–444.

Veljovic, M., Despotovic, S., Stojanovic, M., Pecic, S., Vukosavljevic, P., Belovic, M., & Leskosek-Cukalovic, I. (2015). The fermentation kinetics and physicochemical properties of special beer with addition of prokupac grape variety. *Chemical Industry and Chemical Engineering Quarterly/CICEQ*, *21*(3), 391–397.

Vinson, J. A., Mandarano, M., Hirst, M., Trevithick, J. R., & Bose, P. (2003). Phenol antioxidant quantity and quality in foods: Beers and the effect of two types of beer on an animal model of atherosclerosis. *Journal of Agricultural and Food Chemistry*, *51*(18), 5528–5533.

Williamson, G., & Manach, C. (2005). Bioavailability and bioefficacy of polyphenols in humans. II. Review of 93 intervention studies. *American Journal of Clinical Nutrition*, *81*(1), 243S–255S.

Zhang, K. Z., Deng, K., Luo, H. B., Zhou, J., Wu, Z. Y., & Zhang, W. X. (2013). Antioxidant properties and phenolic profiles of four Chinese Za wines produced from hull-less barley or maize. *Journal of the Institute of Brewing*, *119*(3), 182–190.

Zhao, H., Chen, W., Lu, J., & Zhao, M. (2010). Phenolic profiles and antioxidant activities of commercial beers. *Food Chemistry*, *119*(3), 1150–1158.

8 Comparative Quality Analysis of Different Beers

Beer is a naturally occurring beverage that contains organic acids and vitamins, proteins, hops, water, and little to no fat or calories. Beer has a higher nutritional value than other alcoholic beverages since it contains important nutrients like potassium, magnesium, calcium, and sodium as well as valuable minerals. Beer made from cereals and malt may also help people consume naturally occurring antioxidant components like polyphenols.

More than 3,000 distinct chemicals have been identified in beer, including polyphenols, ions, microorganisms, carbohydrates, proteins, and organic acids, among others. Beer's complexity increases after storage because it may experience chemical changes that harm its flavor, fragrance, and appearance. Being knowledgeable about appropriate analytical procedures for beer evaluation is helpful for academics and brewers because beer is such a widely consumed beverage worldwide.

Brewer's wort, which is made of barley malt, water, and hops, undergoes alcoholic fermentation using yeast. A chemically complex product is produced by various ingredients and brewing process combinations, and it comes in a wide variety of types and styles (Wunderlich & Back, 2009). Beers are primarily categorized as having a top fermentation or high fermentation and a bottom fermentation or low fermentation.

The most popular type of beer, lager, is made through "low" fermentation, which takes place in a cold environment (typically 6 and 15°C). Yeast cells accumulate at the fermenter's bottom after fermentation and are typically removed. In contrast, "high" fermentation, which takes place between 16 and 24°C, results in the production of ale-type beers. During this fermentation, yeast cells rise to the surface of the fermentation media and form a thick film that is typically not completely removed. Different beer styles, including pilsner (the typical American lager), bock, *weizen*, pale and brown ales, *Rauchbier*, and many others, result from changes in the methods of production, ingredient combinations, and processing.

A beer's flavor, aroma, and color are all influenced by the ingredients used in its brewing process; thus, choosing high-quality components is crucial. Brewers generally choose components mostly based on sensory analysis. Brewers could better ensure consistency across batches and create more meaningful ingredient specifications if they conducted a more thorough examination of the primary ingredients before or during the brewing process.

All plant organs contain polyphenolic chemicals, which constitute a crucial component of the human diet. The phenylpropanoid biosynthetic pathway, which also

DOI: 10.1201/b22906-8

yields a wide range of plant phenols, is responsible for their synthesis. Due to their capacity to bind and precipitate macromolecules, polyphenolic compounds have attracted research in recent years.

8.1 pH

The pH of the beer samples ranged from 3.83 to 4.49. The B8 sample was least acidic of all the samples with a pH of 4.49 while the B9 sample was the most acidic with a pH of 3.83. The total acidity of the beer samples was in the range of 0.0957 to 0.2252% tartaric acid equivalent. The B7 sample had the least total acidity of 0.0957±0.0027%, while the B12 sample had the greatest total acidity of 0.2252±0.0%. The pH and total acidity are considered the two most important criteria by the brewing industries, because they strongly influence sanitation and other physiological parameters like color, odor, taste, and biological and chemical stability. The brewing industry usually prefers a pH in a range of 3.90–4.20 for light lager beers, which also plays important role during brewing process that include enzyme effectiveness, hop utilization, and protein coagulation and to monitor yeast activity in clean beer fermentation. Alcoholic beverages from Tanzania were reported to have pH and total acidity in the range of 3.9–5.5 and 0.41–0.062, 0.28–0.38 and 0.06–0.09 g/100 mL, respectively (Tusekwa et al., 2000).

8.2 ORGANIC CONTENT

8.2.1 Carbohydrates

Tracking the concentration of carbohydrates present in wort and beer is very important during brewing. Beer contains approximately 3.3–4.4% carbohydrates, 75 to 80% of which are dextrins, followed by mono- and oligosaccharides, which make up 20 to 30%, and pentosans, which make up 5 to 8%. After fermentation, beer still contains a number of saccharides, including monosaccharides (mostly D-glucose, D-fructose, D-ribose, L-arabinose, D-xylose, and D-galactose in trace amounts), which add to the product's sweetness and make up around 10% of the wort's carbohydrate content. Maltose and sucrose are the main disaccharides, whereas maltotriose, iso-maltose, and raffinose are some important trisaccharides. Studies have shown that these compounds have a number of health advantages, including the prevention of heart disease.

One of the most common methods for the separation and quantitation of carbohydrates in beer is HPLC, which can be coupled with refractive index (RI), ultraviolet (UV), fluorescence (FLD), or mass spectrometric detectors.

In addition to the carbohydrate types of chemicals found in beer, Castellari et al. (2001) suggested a method to quantify organic acids, glycerol, and ethanol using HPLC in a single run. Direct injection of the samples, however, revealed low resolution as a result of interferences. HPLC was connected in series with UV and RI detectors to prevent this. This configuration was intended to lessen retention times and increase separation by limiting matrix interference. With a total analysis duration of 35 to 40 minutes, the HPLC-UV-RI approach allowed for the examination of

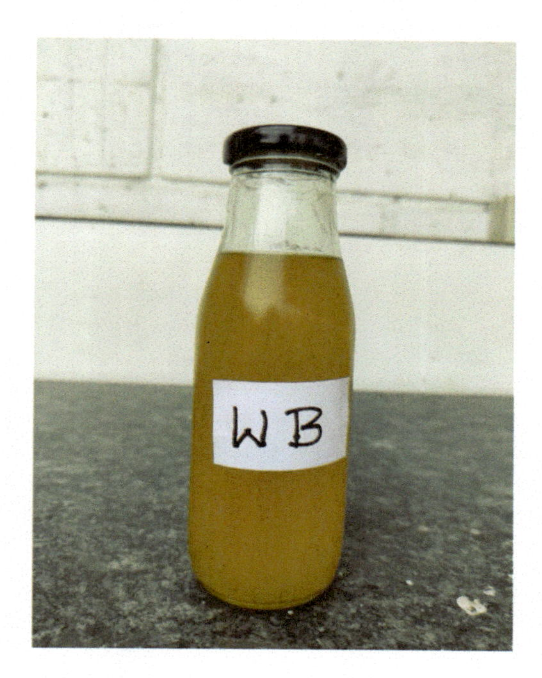

FIGURE 8.1 Wheat Beer

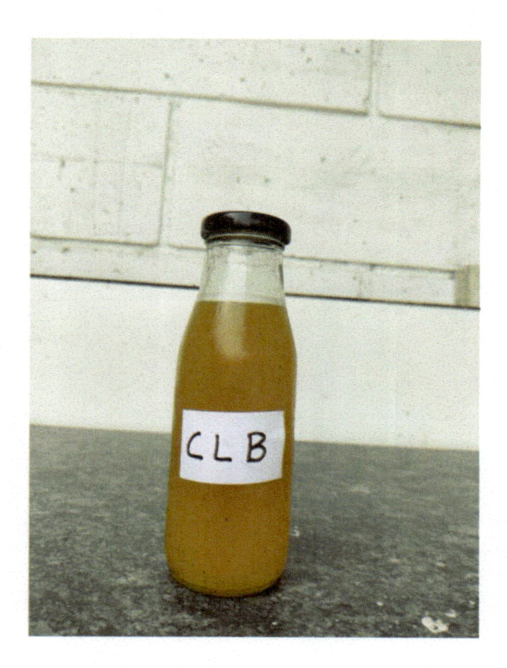

FIGURE 8.2 Lager Beer

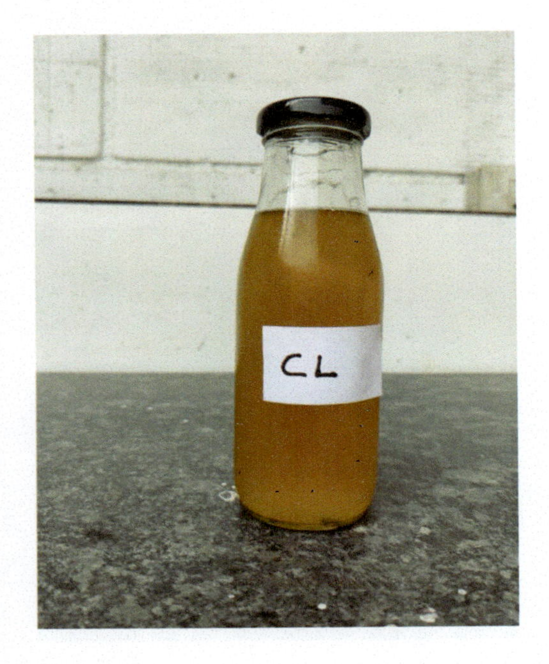

FIGURE 8.3 Lager Beer

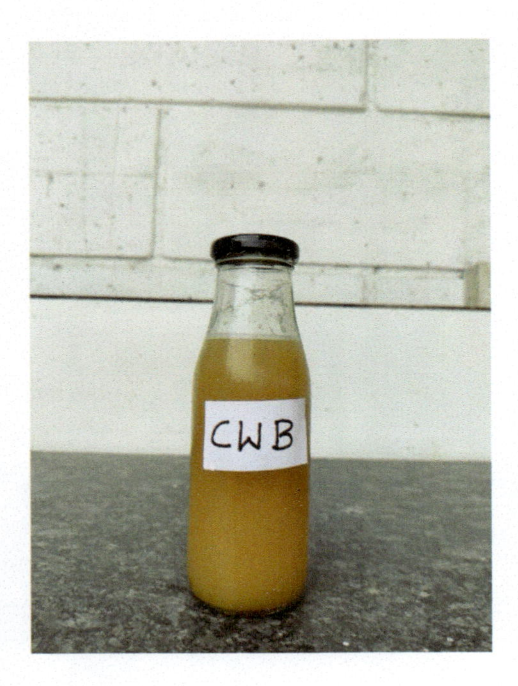

FIGURE 8.4 Wheat Beer

nine different beer constituents. For use in manufacturing and quality control, it has been demonstrated to have adequate accuracy, reproducibility, and limit of quantitation (LOQ). The standard LOQ for carbohydrates by HPLCRI, according to Plata et al. (2013), ranges from 39 to 87 mg/L.

To analyze the changes in the carbohydrate profile during brewing, Rakete and Glomb (2013) developed a novel approach for reversed-phase HPLC coupled to fluorescence or MS detection utilizing 1-naphthylamine for precolumn derivatization with sodium cyanoborohydride. With the right derivatization agent, mass spectrometry's fluorescence activity and sensitivity might be greatly enhanced. Unknown carbohydrates could have their molecular weight and, consequently, their level of polymerization determined by MS detection. Fluorescence was shown to have a limit of detection (LOD) of 1.2M, which is 100 times lower than that of a regularly used technique called fluorophore-assisted carbohydrate electrophoresis (FACE).

Capillary electrophoresis (CE), which offers higher efficiencies, quicker separation times, and less sample preparation than HPLC, is an alternative. The variety of relevant analytes, separation modes, and detectors makes CE a flexible approach. When separating complex carbohydrate samples, CE has an innately high resolving ability, but there are two significant obstacles to be addressed. First, many carbohydrates are difficult to separate by CE because they lack easily ionizable charged functional units. However, by forming complexes with ions like borate and metal cations, the molecules can be changed to charged species "in situ." Assuring their differential electromigration enables their separation in an electric field. The majority of carbohydrates can't absorb light or glow, which makes it difficult for many approaches to detect them. In order to discriminate between the carbohydrates using absorbance or fluorescence detectors, the functional groups (amino and carboxylic acid groups) of the sugar molecules can be marked with UV-absorbing or fluorescent tags.

Carbohydrates can also be analyzed using variations of ion chromatography. This technique has been used to monitor the carbohydrate content throughout the brewing process to determine the extent of fermentation. Fangel et al. (2018) describe the preparation and quantification of β-(1->3) (1->4)-glucan in beer samples using high-performance anion exchange chromatography coupled with pulsed amperometric detection (HPAEC-PAD). The effectiveness and precision of the method were assessed by comparison to carbohydrate microarrays. It was shown that HPAEC-PAD has the ability to distinguish oligosaccharides from β-(1->3) (1->4)-glucan and β-(1->4)-glucan and is suitable for ranking beers based on carbohydrate content. The LOD and LOQ of this method are very low, confirming that it is a selective detection system. Ion-exchange chromatography with pulsed amperometric detection can identify malto oligosaccharides in beer and fermentable sugars in wort.

Ion chromatography variants can also be used to evaluate carbohydrates. This method has been used to gauge the degree of fermentation by keeping an eye on the amount of carbohydrates present during the brewing process. Fangel et al. (2018) utilized high-performance anion exchange chromatography and pulsed amperometric detection (HPAEC-PAD) for quantification of β-(1->3) (1->4)-glucan. The method's efficacy and accuracy were evaluated in comparison to carbohydrate microarrays. It was demonstrated that HPAEC-PAD is useful for classifying beers according to their carbohydrate content since it can identify oligosaccharides from β-(1->3)

(1->4)-glucan and β-(1->4)-glucan. This method's LOD and LOQ are extremely low, indicating that it uses a selective detection approach.

Marques et al. (2017) analyzed various beers that were different in relation to the original gravity (initial sugar content), ranging from 12.01 to 13.9 °P; this is due to the roasting malt levels used in brown porter and Irish red ale beers. This provides darkness to malt, reduces enzymatic activity, and creates worts with less sugar. The appropriateness of the yeast utilized was demonstrated by the apparent attenuation, which ranged from 75.77 to 79.51%. The objective of creating various beer varieties was accomplished because the alcohol, color, and bitterness factors were in line with BJCP (2015) (Strong & England, 2015). The turbidity of the craft beer ranged from 18.35 EBC to 25.77 EBC. This is a wider range than those found in wheat beers (He et al., 2012) but similar to those seen in commercial beers (Steiner et al., 2012). Beer's buttery aroma is caused by vicinal diketones (Liguori et al., 2015). U.S. beers' vicinal diketones were analyzed and ranged from 20 to 100 ppb (Krogerus et al., 2013).

Beer samples had reducing sugar concentrations ranging from 2.682 mg/mL to 0.469 mg/mL. The beer sample containing the highest amount of reducing sugar was B2 (2.682 mg/mL), whereas the lowest value was observed in sample B14 (0.469 mg/mL). Yeast can only utilize a few sugars with lower molecular weights, such as fructose, maltotriose, glucose, maltose, and sucrose. Oligosaccharide cannot be fermented if it contains more than three glucose units. As a result, once the fermentation is allowed to finish, tiny quantities of carbohydrates with lower molecular weights exist in beer (Lehtonen & Hurme, 1994). In some beer styles, the fermentation is stopped early.

The majority of alcohol produced during beer fermentation is related to the synthesis of yeast proteins; which are produced from keto acids. The ethanol percentage ranged from 4.45 to 8.91% volume/volume. The B2 sample had the highest alcohol level at 8.91% by volume, while the B14 sample had the lowest at 4.45% by volume. Many beers have an alcohol concentration that falls between 3 and 6% (v/v). Then, by decarboxylation and reduction, these keto acids are transformed into higher alcohols.

8.2.2 Volatile Aroma Compounds

In addition to ethanol, some by-products like other alcohols, carbonyl compounds, esters, aldehydes, and acids are produced during fermentation. Understanding the type and quantity of the volatile compounds is crucial for the selection of raw materials and yeast strains as well as for quality control as these compounds contribute to the fragrance and flavor character of beer. A widely used method for locating and identifying volatile fragrance molecules is gas chromatography-mass spectrometry (GC-MS). The volatile chemicals must first be removed using headspace (HS) procedures and/or solid phase microextraction (SPME) methods since beer also contains nonvolatile components, and direct infusion into the GC results in contamination. For detecting volatile species in materials with a complex matrix, like beer, headspace extraction is a useful method. The technique is based on collecting the headspace (vapor phase) above the liquid sample in a closed vial and measuring it using a gas chromatograph (GC). The volatile sample is isolated using HS-GC in combination with SPME, considerably minimizing the nonvolatile species' interference. SPME needs less sample preparation and does away with the use of potentially harmful organic solvents.

HS-SPME-GC has been effectively used in a number of beer aroma studies. With the help of optimized HS-SPME-GC-MS, Cajka et al. (2010) observed relatively good repeatability of peak height measurements within a series of ten consecutive analyses of beer for 45 selected volatile compounds. Several volatile indicators were chosen and categorized in accordance with classes of alcohols, aldehydes, ketones, esters, carboxylic acids, ethers, and other substances after GC profiles were examined. Different techniques in which each group altered the beer profile were demonstrated.

Esters have a fruity flavor and have been demonstrated to affect the harmony of the flavors in a dish. Higher alcohols function as the direct antecedents of the more flavor-active esters, and they also add to the strong aroma and flavor of beer. Aldehydes and ketones have been found to closely correlate with the formation of stale flavors during storage. Carboxylic acids can be a part of a variety of smells, including fruity, cheesy, bitter, or rotten. The creation of sweeter scents like caramelized sugar and almond is also influenced by ethers.

Using a flame ionization detector is another way to carry out this procedure (FID). Jiao et al. (2021) were successful in obtaining the chromatographic fingerprint of the flavor in diverse beer samples using HS-SPME-GC-FID. Twenty-eight beer samples were categorized by type, taste, and brewery after applying principal component analysis (PCA) and hierarchal clustering analysis (HCA) to analyze the GC data. Charry-Parra et al. (2011) reported that the HS-SPME-GC-FID technique is a straightforward one that may be utilized for quality control under typical brewery production settings.

8.2.3 Vicinal Diketones

Molecules possessing two ketone groups on nearby (vicinal) carbon atoms are known as vicinal diketones (VDKs). The two most frequent ones, 2,3-butanedione (commonly known as diacetyl) and 2,3-pentanedione, which provide off tastes associated with lager degradation, are detected in beer. VDKs are created during fermentation, but they are not created by the yeast directly; rather, they are created through a long-chain reaction. The precursors acetolactate and aceto hydroxybutyrate are ejected by yeast cells during the production of valine and isoleucine; they then go through oxidative decarboxylation to create diacetyl and pentanedione, respectively. Diacetyl has distinct flavors like sweet butter, caramel, and butterscotch, whereas pentanedione gives the beer a honey-like flavor. Tian discovered that the ratio of VDKs (diacetyl/pentanedione) also produced off odors and indicated the level of contamination in beer. In samples that were significantly contaminated by bacteria during fermentation, pentanedione content (g/L) was decreased while a notable rise in diacetyl was noted at the same time. As a result, it was established that a "normal" beer had a ratio of about one, whereas contaminated beers had a ratio of more than one. The measurement of these two VDKs should be significant to the brewing industry because they are utilized as target analytes to regulate beer quality.

VDKs should be prepared for examination using HS-SPME-GC as with volatile aroma chemicals. By allowing simultaneous sampling, extraction, pre-concentration, and insertion of analytes into the GC in a single step, HS-SPME is a solvent-free sample preparation approach that increases the lifespan of the column and prevents contamination. There are several detectors that can be employed, including MS, FID, and electron capture detectors (ECD). In order to measure VDKs in beer, Hernandes et al. (2019) employed HS-SPME-GC-MS, which showed great sensitivity and was helpful for quality control. Although ECD is used to identify substances with high electron affinities, such as pentanedione and diacetyl, which have the capacity to grab electrons, it may be more appropriate for VDK analysis than MS or FID. The analyte concentration is proportional to the degree of electron capture and can be identified by the peak area in a chromatogram because electron capture causes the current between the anode and cathode of the detector to decrease. Numerous times, HS-SPME-GC-ECD has been utilized successfully to identify VDKs. This detection technique was demonstrated to be very sensitive, accurate, selective, and precise, even for trace analysis. However, challenges like the ECD's constrained linear dynamic range must be resolved (Alves et al., 2020).

8.2.4 Organic Acids

Both yeast fermentation and bacterial fermentation produce organic acids as their by-products. These acids play a crucial role in the taste profile, although bacterial fermentation can result in the introduction of a sour flavor. This flavor may be intended when making sour beers, or it may be inadvertent as a result of spoiling. Depending on the yeast strain and brewing technique employed, organic acids produced during fermentation will differ in kind and quantity. Beer's pH and flavor (sour, tart, acidic) are influenced by organic acids, which also have advantageous physiological benefits, including lowering uric acid. By preventing the growth of some spoilage bacteria like *Salmonella*, the presence of these acids may also aid in extending the beer's shelf life. Due to its speed, stability, and ease of sample preparation, high-performance liquid chromatography (HPLC) is a well-liked method for analyzing organic acids. The total amount of organic acids found in four distinct beer samples was found to range between 451 mg/L and 712 mg/L using HPLC, according to Montanari et al. (1999).

There were several common organic acids discovered, with lactic acid often having the greatest concentration. These also included tartaric, malic, acetic, citric, and succinic acids. The approach was demonstrated to operate adequately when used in the analysis of fruits and juices, which have a lot of the same organic acids as beer.

For instance, the analytical figures of merit for the determination of tartaric acid included the following: Linearity (R2) of > 0.999, relative standard deviation (RSD) values between 0.38 and 1.28% for repeatability and 0.85 to 1.59% for reproducibility, a LOD of 0.72 g/mL and a LOQ of 2.40 g/mL, and a LOD of 0.72 g/mL and a LOQ of 2.

However, the insufficient selectivity and sensitivity offered by traditional liquid chromatographic detectors has hampered the capacity of HPLC to identify low quantities of organic acids in beer. Due to the fact that organic acids lack strong chromophores or fluorophores, this also applies to absorbance and fluorescence detectors.

Chemiluminescence (CL) and photochemical reactions are combined in a unique post-column reaction detection method developed by Perez-Ruiz et al. (2004) to analyze various acids. In the absence of a light source, noise is reduced, Rayleigh and Raman scattering are eliminated, and photon detectors may operate at high gain to increase the signal-to-noise ratio. This makes CL detection exceedingly sensitive. Due to their selectivity and specificity, several photochemical processes have been used as post-column detection techniques in liquid chromatography.

Beer chromatograms were compared using photochemical-CL detection and absorbance detection, and it was shown that the absorbance chromatogram was much more complicated, had poorly formed peaks, and had an unstable baseline. The authors discovered lactic acid (559–631 mg/L), malic acid (40–68 mg/L), tartaric acid (0–24 mg/L), oxalic acid (12–25 mg/L), and citric acid (74–202 mg/L) with great sensitivity and selectivity using the combined HPLC-photochemical-CL detection method on four distinct beers.

8.2.5 Iso-α-Acids

The unique bitterness present in beer is due the α-acids (humulones) and β-acids (lupulones) present in hops. Wort boiling leads to chemical conversion of α-acids to iso-α-acids (isomerization) via an acylon-type ring contraction. About 80% of the bitter flavor in beer comes from iso-acids, whose concentrations range from 15 mg/L in standard American lagers to approximately 100 mg/L in really bitter English ales.

The quantity of isomerization and bitterness are inversely correlated and heavily influenced by the hop strain and duration of boiling. Iso-acids are interesting because of their impact on foam stability and their bacteriostatic properties, in addition to their bitterness. Additionally, it has been reported that these acids may improve cognitive decline (dementia) brought on by high-fat diets and decrease the development of liver tumors in mice.

The most popular method for determining beer bitterness is based on measuring the UV absorbance of an iso-octane extract of acidified beer at 275 nm. Lead conductance, automated discrete photometry, electric tongue, and other techniques are also often used. These techniques, however, can be laborious, difficult, and general. As a result, HPLC has been used more often to determine iso-α-acids quantitatively.

There are various benefits of using an improved HPLC approach to iso-α-acids. For instance, it can show variations in the isomerization kinetics of individual α-acids, variations in the behavior of individual iso-α-acids in response to foam portioning, and variations in the behavior of individual α-acids during beer storage. The use of this method has certain drawbacks as well. During the chromatographic run, iso-acids frequently interact with trace metals, which has been found to result in poor analyte recovery and resolution. The use of top-notch solvents and a completely demineralized column can prevent these problems.

8.2.6 Polyphenols and Antioxidant Activity

Polyphenols belong to a group of easily oxidizable substances that have the potential to act as antioxidants by stopping the oxidation of other molecules. Additionally, polyphenols can affect the beer's color, flavor (bitterness, astringency, and harshness), and colloidal stability. The majority of the polyphenols (roughly 70%) come from the malt, while the remaining approximately 30% come from the hops, with the precise percentage dependent on the hop strain and the stage of addition. Belonging to the groups of simple phenols, benzoic and cinnamic acid derivatives, coumarins, catechins, (prenylated) chalcones, and flavonoids, phenolic components of beer come in a wide range of structural configurations.

Flavan-3-ols and their condensed derivatives, the proanthocyanidins, which have been demonstrated to affect the colloidal stability, are some typical phenolic elements found in beer. Due to the complexation of proteins and polyphenols in beer, which results in the development of finely distributed precipitates, this stability is the tendency of beer to generate haze. Cold filtration or adsorptive resins like polyvinylpyrrolidone can be employed to eliminate the unwelcome haziness brought on by the interactions between the polyphenol and the proteins (PVPP). Although removing polyphenols increases the shelf life of beer in terms of haze formation, PVPP is not selective for doing so and may therefore result in the loss of taste-active polyphenols as well.

Analysis of the total polyphenol content (TPC) is necessary to avoid the creation of unwelcome haze. Because of the low cost, simplicity of use, and speed of analysis, colorimetric reactions in combination with UV-Vis spectrophotometric techniques are frequently employed for total polyphenol analyses. The Folin-Ciocalteu reagent, which is a combination of tungstate and molybdate, is used to oxidize polyphenolic compounds in an alkaline medium to produce a colored complex that can be measured spectrophotometrically. This procedure is a well-established technique for measuring TPC. Tannic acid was proven to have superior recovery rates and less interference from the sample than gallic acid, which was employed as the calibration curve reference chemical in the majority of these experiments. This approach has the disadvantage of using phosphotungstic or phosphomolybdic acids, which produce trash that cannot be recycled. Additionally, the beer sample may contain certain reducing agents that might affect the reagent, such as citric acid, sulfites, or simple sugars. The tests' findings demonstrated that TPC differed greatly depending on the kind of beer. According to Piazzon et al., the tendency is as follows: dealcoholized lager, pilsner, wheat beer, ale, abbey, and bock. Additionally, it was shown that more hoppy beers had greater polyphenol content, which was to be expected given that hops are the source of certain polyphenols.

Phenolic compounds are by far the most common dietary antioxidants in the average human diet. An important group of these found in beer are the flavan-3-ols, which behave as antioxidants via scavenging of free radicals and chelate transition metals, as well as mediating and inhibiting enzyme activity. When comparing beers with varying antioxidant activity, those which were more abundant in phenolic antioxidants exhibited higher quality in terms of foamability and heat and oxidative stability, as well as a longer shelf life. The shelf life is believed to be increased due to the antioxidants counteracting the autoxidative mechanisms of the iso-α-acids. It has also been reported that the antioxidant content of beer has positive health effects in humans when consumed in moderation, such as increasing the plasma antioxidant and anticoagulant activities and improving plasma lipid levels.

The antioxidant activity of beer polyphenols has been monitored using a variety of techniques. To identify the important antioxidants in pilsner-style beer, Spreng and Hofmann (2018) used activity-guided fractionation in conjunction with oxygen radical absorbance capacity (ORAC), hydrogen peroxide scavenging (HPS), and linoleic acid (LA) tests. The structural identification of 31 antioxidants was made possible by LC-TOF-MS investigations that were followed by 1D/2D NMR spectroscopy tests. This was the first research to demonstrate that the highest levels of antioxidant activity in beer were displayed by hordatines, saponarin, and quercetin-3-O-β-D-(6"-O-malonyl) glucoside. The ferric reducing antioxidant power (FRAP) test, which gauges a sample's antioxidant capacity by watching a ferric tripyridyl triazine complex's transformation into its colored, ferrous form in the presence of antioxidants, is another useful assay. In order to assess the antioxidant activity of seven distinct types of beers, five samples of various brands were utilized in the FRAP experiment by Piazzon et al. Results revealed a substantial association ($r = 0.92$) between antioxidant activity as evaluated by the FRAP test and TPC as determined by the Folin-Ciocalteu technique, and a very similar pattern in beer type was identified: dealcoholized pilsner, lager, wheat, ale, abbey, and bock. The activity varied from 1,525 mol/L for dealcoholized beer to 4,663 mol/L for bock beers and was expressed as micromoles of Fe^{2+} per liter of beer. The ferric tripyridyl triazine reduction might be brought on by any substance with an appropriate redox potential, which is one drawback of the FRAP test. Procedures for assay-guided fractionation frequently take a long time.

Recent years have seen the development of a number of sensitive post column HPLC techniques for antioxidant analysis, which are intended to test for antioxidant activity more quickly and directly than conventional bulk assays. Beer polyphenols may be separated using HPLC using a technique known as liquid chromatography-antioxidant (LC-AOx), and the antioxidant contribution of each component can then be assessed. The 2,2′-azinobis (3-ethylbenzothiazoline-6-sulfonic acid) radical cation (ABTS+), which exhibits a drop in absorbance at 734 nm after reacting with a reducing agent, is a stable model free-radical system that is needed for this approach. Comparing this strategy to conventional HPLC with UV detection, reactive antioxidants may show to be more sensitive to it. As the brewing process progressed, Leitao et al. used LC-AOx followed by UV-Vis detection to monitor the antioxidant activity of beer extracts (brewing, boiling, and fermentation). It was observed that after hopping and fermentation, the polyphenolic content increased by three times while the overall antioxidant activity remained constant. The authors claimed that the presence of ethanol after fermentation improved chemical extraction since they were unable to identify polyphenol content in hop extracts using the LC-AOx technique.

Moura-Nunes et al. (2016) analyzed and compared the phenolic compounds in Brazilian beer of different types and styles. Chemometrics were also applied for modeling beer's antioxidant capacity as a function of its physicochemical attributes (density, refractive index, bitterness, and ethanol content). PCA was used to analyze samples ($n = 29$), dividing them into five groups based on characteristics like ethanol content and bitterness. In comparison to Groups I (non-alcoholic beers) and II, Group V (alcoholic beers with very high bitterness) generally displayed higher refractive index, bitterness, ethanol, and phenolic content (alcoholic beers with low bitterness).

Brazilian beers had a different phenolic profile from European beers, with higher gallic acid concentrations (0.5–14.7 mg/L) and lower ferulic acid concentrations

(0.2–1.8 mg/L). By using PLS, the ethanol content and density, bitterness, and refractive index values of beer could be used to predict its antioxidant capacity, which was determined using the FRAP assay. It was observed that commercial beers showed physicochemical attributes in accordance with international regulations. It was also observed that Brazilian beers exhibited almost similar phenolic content and antioxidant activity to beers elsewhere in world. Gallic acid content was higher, and ferulic acid content was lower in Brazilian beer's phenolic profiles.

Nardini and Garaguso (2020) analyzed different fruit beers for total polyphenol and flavonoid content, phenolic profile by using HPLC, and antioxidant activity. Cherry, raspberry, peach, apricot, grape, plum, orange, and apple were used to produce fruit beers and added at the time of fermentation. In comparison to traditional non-fruit beers, most of the fruit beers had significantly higher levels of antioxidant activity, total polyphenols, and flavonoids. The highest values are found in cherry beers, followed by grape, plum, and orange beers. All the fruit beers under investigation showed enrichment in their catechin and quercetin content. Most of the fruit beers also contained myricetin and resveratrol and were found to contain more chlorogenic, neochlorogenic, p-coumaric, and caffeic acids than conventional beers. Results demonstrated that the addition of fruits during the fermentation process significantly increased the antioxidant activity of beer and enhanced both the qualitative and quantitative phenolic profile.

Oroian et al. (2016) evaluated the polyphenol content and antioxidant activity of ten different beers purchased from a local market in Romania. The Folin-Ciocalteu method was used to determine the polyphenol content of the beer samples. The total polyphenol concentration of the ten beer samples under study varied significantly, from 61.40 mg GAE/L for Landbier to 361.40 mg GAE/L for Skol beer. It was observed that polyphenol concentration was highest in Skol then followed by Suceava > Ursus > Timisoreana > Tuborg > Silva bruna > Ursus bruna > Gauloise > Guinness > Landbier. Beers like Guinness, Gauloise, and Suceava had significant levels of polyphenol (>100 mg GAE/L). Using the DPPH assay, the antioxidant capacity of the beer samples was determined. A UV-VIS spectrophotometer was used to implement the two methods. All the beer samples had robust DPPH radical activity throughout the concentration test. The range of PI percent values is 10.24 to 33.68%. The highest antioxidant activity was observed in Tuborg beer and lowest in Landbier among all the samples. It was demonstrated that the brewing technique and raw ingredients had a substantial impact on the DPPH radical activity of the samples.

Marques et al. (2017) observed considerable levels of phenolics, and the values ranged from 448.57 to 531.30 mg GAE/L. The total values of phenolic compounds were lower than those published by Piazzon et al. (2010) (875 mg GAE/L), but higher than those reported by Zhao et al. (2010), which ranged from 152.01 to 339.12 mg GAE/L. Beers with a high original gravity and a dark hue, which tend to enhance the value of phenolic chemicals, can be used to explain this divergence (Piazzon et al., 2010). Lipid oxidation is caused by the hydrogen free radical's capacity to scavenge other radicals, particularly hydroperoxide radicals (Zhao et al., 2013). The ability of the beers to suppress free radicals ranged from 29.4 to 48.5%. These percentages are in line with those seen in Brazilian commercial beers, which Granato et al. (2011) found to range from 4.75 to 59.98%.

According to Zhao et al. (2010), beers with a high caffeic acid content are those with the strongest radical scavenging activity, which prevents lipid oxidation, and the beer brown porter demonstrated the greatest inhibitory ability (Aron et al., 2010). In the phenolic profile of beers, caffeic acid was observed in the greatest concentration (9.05 mg/L).

The quantity of phenolic acids in different beers varies due to variation in their brewing steps, in particular filtering and clarifying, which affect the composition (Gorjanovic et al., 2010). The raw materials used to manufacture beer also influence the final product, such as phenolic acids profile. The malt and hops vary greatly in polyphenols content due to cultivation region, crop handling, and processing (Piazzon et al., 2010; Vanderhaegen et al., 2006). Beer has a high concentration of bioactive chemicals and a low alcohol content. Studies have indicated that moderate beer intake in adults (one to three doses per day) is linked to a healthy cardiovascular system, which results in a 30–40% reduction in coronary disease compared to non-drinkers (Piazzon et al., 2010).

8.2.7 Mycotoxins

Mycotoxins, which are poisonous secondary metabolites produced by fungi, can have both immediate and long-term impacts on both people and animals. To make sure the concentrations are within permissible levels, it is advised to measure the amount in finished beer in addition to testing the barley for mycotoxins.

Deoxynivalenol (DON) and zearalenone (ZEN) have maximum allowable concentrations in cereal-based products (like beer) of 750 g/L and 75 g/L, respectively, under current European mycotoxins standards. The FDA's recommended amount of DON in grain by-products for human consumption as of 2010 is 1 mg/L. Beer was examined for the presence of mycotoxins using HPLC-UV at 218 nm by Basalekou et al. (2022). The technique was demonstrated to have an LOD of 1.3 g/L and acceptable recovery and reproducibility ranges (precision, RSD). In this investigation, DON was found in 83% of the samples, with an average content of 9.0–12.7 g/L, which is considered low enough to be safe (Bryła et al., 2018).

Enzyme immunoassays are fast screening techniques that may be used as a secondary tool to examine for the presence of mycotoxins. This method was utilized by Bauer et al. (2016) to examine the amounts of DON and ZEN as well as ergot alkaloids and alternariol (AOH) in German beers. This approach has the advantage that just DON needs to be extracted in order to attain a sensitive LOD and lower the minimum sample dilution factor. Only dilution and pH correction were required for the remaining samples. The ergot alkaloid detection limits (measured as ergometrine equivalents) were 0.06 g/L, ergot alkaloids (measured as 2.1 g/L DON), 0.14 g/L ZEN, and 0.18 g/L AOH. Results revealed that 75% of beer samples contained DON, 93% of samples tested positive for ergot alkaloids, and all samples tested positive for ZEN and AOH. The conclusion was reached that beer is not a significant source of intake of these toxins despite the frequency of occurrence since concentrations of all the analytes were below the daily tolerated consumption for the European Union. Even while it appears that mycotoxins are present in the majority of beers at acceptably low levels, analysis is nevertheless advised to validate this.

8.3 INORGANIC CONTENT

8.3.1 Total SO_2

The majority of the sulfur dioxide (SO_2) in beer comes from the metabolism of the yeast or any exogenous sulfite that is added prior to packing. In order to create hydroxysulfonates, which are not flavor active and hence raise the flavor threshold of the carbonyls that give beer its stale, disagreeable flavors, SO_2 reacts with carbonyl molecules (often aldehydes) to enhance flavor stability. At high quantities, SO_2 also functions as an antibacterial and antioxidant.

A tiny percentage of people do, however, have sulfite sensitivity, which has a wide range of dermatological, pulmonary, gastrointestinal, and cardiovascular symptoms as side effects. SO_2 levels must be kept under control to prevent these harmful impacts on human health. According to US and EU rules, alcoholic drinks must label their total SO_2 concentration if it is identified at a level of 10 mg/L or greater.

The American Society of Brewing Chemists (ASBC) recommends colorimetric analysis as one of the most popular methods for determining total SO_2 in foods and drinks. With this technique, bound SO_2 is first hydrolyzed with an alkali solution, and then after approximately 30 minutes, SO_2, p-rosaniline, and formaldehyde react to produce a colorful solution (Stewart et al., 2017).

At 550 nm, the complex's absorbance may be seen. Although this technique has been widely utilized because of its accuracy and capacity to measure both free and total SO_2, the entire process is time consuming and necessitates handling the potentially cancer-causing compound p-rosaniline. By modifying a procedure utilizing flow injection analysis (FIA), these problems can be minimized.

In order to liberate bound sulfites before injection, this method entails putting the beer sample into a mixing chamber with sodium hydroxide (NaOH). In order to reduce the pH and transform the equilibrium products already present into gaseous sulfur dioxide, which is separated by diffusion over a gas permeable membrane, sulfuric acid is injected. The colorful product is then produced by the SO_2 reacting with p-rosaniline and formaldehyde and is quantified using a spectrophotometer. Using the merging zones approach, the p-rosaniline is delivered into the system in a way that decreases its consumption by introducing just the quantity needed for the reaction, as opposed to a continuous flow through the manifold.

The FIA system has several advantages over the conventional method, including the absence of sample preparation requirements, greater sampling rates, accurate and exact findings, and a tenfold decrease in p-rosaniline consumption. Beer's total and free SO_2 concentrations have been determined using voltammetric techniques as well. Beer samples are diluted in an alkaline solution with NaOH in the first stage, which causes adducts between SO_2 and carbonyls to disintegrate and turns hydrogen sulfite into sulfite. Nitrogen is used to remove the volatile aldehydes (mostly acetaldehyde) from the sample, which are then collected in the proper electrolyte trapping solution, derivatized with hydrazine, and measured voltammetrically. The remaining beer sample is acidified to completely transform all the sulfite into SO_2, which is then transported by nitrogen gas into a trapping solution.

The total SO_2 concentration is then calculated using voltammetry. Since the acetaldehyde-hydrogen sulfite adduct is quite stable and accounts for around 95% of all the aldehydes in beer, the free SO_2 concentration may be determined by subtracting the total SO_2 concentration from the acetaldehyde concentration. With respect to the overall SO_2 concentrations commonly seen in beer, our approach revealed an RSD of around 2.1%. Voltammetric measurements appear to be in agreement with the results of the p-rosaniline reference technique, with the benefit of avoiding the use of hazardous reagents (p-rosaniline) and producing more precise and accurate results.

8.3.2 Ions

Metal cations, trace metals, and anions are inorganic substances that are present in beer and have an impact on the clarity and salty flavor of the beverage. These substances can come from a variety of sources, including the raw ingredients (often malt), brewing building materials, or the processing and packaging of the completed beer. Most brewing water is deionized to standardize the quality before putting back the necessary ions. Inorganic component concentrations typically range from 0.5–2 g/L.

The two ions of greatest relevance are chloride and sulfate because chloride gives flavors a mellower, fuller quality while sulfate makes a beer more arid tasting. Nitrate, phosphate, iron, copper, zinc, manganese, nickel, and aluminum are some additional frequently occurring ions. Beer's inorganic ions can also be identified using atomic emission spectrometry with inductively coupled plasma (ICP-AES); however, inorganic ion analysis is commonly done via ion chromatography (IC) or capillary electrophoresis (CE).

When it was initially developed in 1975, ion chromatography was only used to measure inorganic ions; however, it has since been expanded to measure organic ions, various separation techniques (such as ion exclusion), simultaneous separation of anions and cations, and a variety of detectors. It is frequently used to identify different inorganic ions in alcoholic drinks, including beer, wine, and vodka. For the purpose of determining the cations in beer, Zeng et al. (2006) effectively used IC with acidified aqueous mobile phases and non-suppressed conductivity detection. For the targeted ions, this method demonstrated acceptable sensitivity, detection limits, and repeatability. This method's ability to inject the beer samples instantly after dilution without any additional preparation was one of its benefits. Aluminum in beer may be examined using IC, as well as anions including chloride, sulfate, nitrate, and phosphate.

For the examination of inorganic anions in four different varieties of beer, Klampfl looked into the usage of CZE outfitted with a conductivity detector in series with a fixed-wavelength UV detector operating at 254 nm. The optimal detection technique for each type of analyte was used to conduct quantitation employing both detectors at once.

For instance, phosphate favored UV detection, whereas chloride and sulfate were better suited for conductivity detection. This method produced good limits of detection for the target analytes, with RSD values between 0.5 and 6.6% and ranges from 0.02 mg/L for chloride to 0.41 mg/L for phosphate. It simply took dilution and 15 minutes of degassing to prepare the sample. For the simultaneous detection of inorganic and organic anions, amino acids, and carbohydrates in pineapple and soy sauce samples, CZE was demonstrated to be a straightforward and reliable technique. This strategy has potential for beer analysis as well.

Both IC and CE were determined to have certain benefits over one another when compared. While there are more than enough commercially available stationary phases for IC, CE selectivity depends on the analytes' electrophoretic mobilities and is hence far more challenging to manage. In everyday situations (direct injection), IC is also far more sensitive and may reach RSD (precision) of 1% or less, whereas CE's RSD is normally between 3 and 5%. The speed of analysis, cost of consumables, and separation efficiency (which is 50 times more than that of IC) are among areas in which CE shines. Despite their differences, these approaches' separation selectivities complement one another in that a sample separation that is challenging with one is frequently rather simple with the other. Combining the two methods has the advantages of reducing interferences from other ions and confirming peak identification. Capillary electrophoresis is becoming increasingly widely used and may eventually completely replace ion chromatography (IC), despite the fact that IC is an older and more advanced technology.

The inorganic compounds found in beer are metal cations, trace metals, and anions, which influence the drink's clarity and salty taste. These compounds can originate from several places, such as the raw materials (usually malt, since most brewing water is deionized to standardize the quality before adding back the requisite ions), brewing construction materials, or the processing and packing of the finished beer. Concentrations of inorganic components generally range from 0.5–2 g/L.

Chloride and sulfate are the ions of highest interest, as chloride provides mellowing and fullness to the flavor while sulfate enhances the dry character of a beer. Some other commonly found ions include nitrate, phosphate, iron, copper, zinc, manganese, nickel, and aluminum. Inorganic ion analysis is typically performed by ion chromatography (IC) or capillary electrophoresis (CE), although atomic emission spectrometry with inductively coupled plasma (ICP-AES) can also be used to determine the inorganic ions in beer.

Ion chromatography was used specifically for the determination of inorganic ions when it was first introduced in 1975, but its use later broadened to include organic ions, other separation methods (e.g., ion exclusion), simultaneous separation of anions and cations, and a variety of detectors. It has been used extensively for the determination of various inorganic ions in alcoholic beverages such as beer, wine, and vodka.

Zeng et al. (2006) successfully applied IC with acidified aqueous mobile phases and non-suppressed conductivity detection for the determination of cations in beer. This technique showed satisfactory sensitivity, detection limits, and reproducibility for the ions of interest. One advantage of this method was that it allowed the beer samples to be injected directly after dilution with no other preparation. IC is useful for analyzing aluminum in beer, as well as anions such as chloride, sulfate, nitrate, and phosphate.

8.4 BIOLOGICAL

8.4.1 Bacteria

One of the oldest styles of sour beer still being made is lambic, which has been the subject of research on bacterial analysis. Although lambic beers are only produced in Belgium, sour beers in general are increasingly gaining popularity around the world. For instance, American craft brewers have begun producing American coolship ales by imitating the production process for lambic beer. These beers' sour flavor is principally caused by the metabolism of different yeasts, lactic acid bacteria (LAB), and acetic acid bacteria (AAB). The undesirable impacts of these bacteria, however, include beer deterioration, turbidity, acidity, and bad tastes.

Brewers must thus characterize beer spoilage microorganisms in order to ensure product quality. Prior microbiological research on beers solely employed phenotypic identification approaches, which current studies have shown to be insufficient for the species-level identification of yeasts, LAB, and AAB due to their lack of taxonomic precision.

MALDI-TOF-MS is a new option for categorizing bacteria in beer since it can distinguish between organisms at the genus, species, or strain level. By comparing the MALDI-TOF-MS spectra acquired from straightforward microbial mixes and cultivated bacterial cells to a library of known spectral fingerprints derived from intact bacterial cells, studies have successfully identified bacterial cells (Lay, 2000). As an alternative, MALDI may desorb proteins from whole cells of microorganisms to produce spectra with distinct indicators that can be compared to a protein database. Wieme et al. (2014) built a comprehensive database of more than 4,200 mass spectra, comprising duplicates produced from AAB and LAB, spanning a total of 52 species, cultivated on at least three growth conditions, for the identification of beer-spoilage bacteria by MALDI-TOF-MS.

The ruined beer samples had insufficient bacterial cells to enable direct detection and classification using MALDI855 TOF-MS; as a result, enrichment and separation of the germs were required before analysis. With the use of protein coding gene sequence analysis, the obtained identifications were confirmed. Of the collected isolates from samples of damaged beer, 327 of the 348 were easily identified as being different species according to peak-based numerical analysis of the MALDI spectra (which accounted for 94% of the total isolates).

This method was shown to be suitable for regular microbiological quality monitoring in the brewing sector because of the cheap consumable cost, high throughput, and precise identification of the bacteria. Cheaper alternatives would be preferable because a MALDI-TOF instrument's high initial cost and ongoing maintenance expenses would be prohibitive for small and medium-size brewers. Spitaels et al. (2014) provided a description of variations of MALDI-TOF-MS utilized, particularly for the bacterial investigation of lambic sour beers.

Fatty acids, which are crucial elements of bacterial cell membranes, can be used as another alternative for microbiological examination. Similar to protein profiles, fatty acid profiles differ among bacterial species and can be used to identify them by cross-referencing against a database. A commercially accessible library called the Microbial Identification System (MIS), created by Microbial ID (MIDI, Newark,

DE, USA), is frequently used to identify bacteria by their fatty acid profiles. In most cases, fatty acids are recognized and measured using GC in conjunction with either MS or FID detectors. A recently created method called GC-VUV can deconvolve coeluting peaks by overlapping absorption spectra and offers information equivalent to that of GC-MS, which is useful for complicated beer samples. Santos et al. (2018) identified and distinguished environmental bacteria based on their fatty acid profiles using GC-VUV to detect bacterium fatty acid methyl esters (FAMEs). Santos et al. (2018) also discussed comparison research in which bacteria in water samples were examined for their protein and fatty acid compositions using GC-VUV and MALDI-TOF-MS as a measure of environmental stress. The two techniques were shown to be complementing instruments for environmental analysis.

Although no studies using GC-VUV for bacterial analysis in beer have been discovered, it looks like an intriguing area for future research. Brewers might also wish to quantify the bacteria in their beer in addition to identifying the germs. Combining next-generation sequencing (NGS) and a quantitative polymerase chain reaction (qPCR) test is a promising approach for studying bacterial populations. When Takahashi et al. employed NGS-qPCR to monitor the total numbers of bacteria during fermentation and maturation, they discovered that the populations in beer samples varied between around 103 and 104 cells/mL. Additionally, they discovered that barley's microbial community changes during the malting process and that malt has a higher concentration of bacteria than does barley. In a different investigation, Takahashi et al. (2015) used NGS-qPCR to measure the cell densities of LAB and AAB in 37 samples of craft beer. When the outcomes of this investigation were compared to those of species-specific qPCR, a more well-known technique, they were shown to be reliable. Accordingly, this method seems useful for examining bacterial populations in beer based on the density of LAB and AAB cells.

8.5 FATTY ACIDS

The raw ingredients (malt and hops) and mashing process, as well as yeast metabolism and maturation, all have an impact on the fatty acid composition of beer. Beer quality may be assessed using fatty acid content in addition to bacterial analysis. Fatty acids can harm the flavor of beer even when they are just tiny components, such as staling. Rancid or goaty taste traits are caused by medium-chain fatty acids such hexanoic, octanoic, and decanoic acids. Furthermore, due to their oxidative breakdown, long-chain unsaturated fatty acids like linoleic and linolenic acids may cause the development of an ageing flavor, and an unanticipated rise in their content, along with poor storage conditions, may result in an unfavorable stale flavor. Fatty acids and excessive foaming volume also have an intriguing link. Unsaturated fatty acids have been shown to reduce the amount of spontaneous over-foaming, but saturated fatty acids are known to encourage gushing. An appropriate and trustworthy method for fatty acid analysis is desired due to their influence on numerous elements of beer quality.

Gas chromatography, which has been employed since the 1960s to analyze the changes in beer's volatile components during storage, is often used to quantify fatty acids, as was mentioned in the preceding section. Both MS and FID detection are allowed. These GC methods can make use of a variety of sample preparation methods, which include an essential extraction phase that frequently requires complicated operations.

Techniques like liquid-liquid extraction and steam distillation, which take a lot of time and require a lot of work, were utilized in earlier research. Liquid-liquid extraction also has issues with emulsion formation and needs a lot of organic solvents, which might result in analyte losses. Modern methods rely on solid-phase extraction techniques like stir bar sorptive extraction (SBSE) and solid-phase microextraction (SPME), which are often quicker and require fewer organic solvents overall, resulting in higher recovery and high repeatability. Using a GC-FID approach with liquid-liquid cartridge extraction and SPE purification to prevent emulsion formation and promote the effective extraction of fatty acids present in low concentrations, Bravi et al. (2017) quantitatively measured the fatty acids in beer. However, the process of preparing the sample was complicated by the need to derivatize the fatty acids to their methyl esters (FAMEs) before injecting them into the GC.

Nevertheless, this is a reasonably simple, widely used, and quantifiable approach. Unsaturated oleic and linoleic acids were shown to be the most representative fatty acids on average, which should prevent excessive foaming. The technique was demonstrated to be adaptable to a variety of fatty acids in various beer samples, making it an appropriate option for this kind of study.

8.6 PESTICIDES

Insects and microbiological diseases can damage the grains and hops used in brewing, including hop aphids and two-spotted spider mites. Different mixtures of insecticides are frequently used at numerous phases of cultivation and post-harvest storage to avoid crop damage caused by these pests. Although these pesticides are essential for crop protection, they could get into the beer during brewing and endanger the drinker. Having a thorough approach to identifying the many types of chemicals employed, including glyphosate, glufosinate, chlorfenapyr, quinoxyfen, and fenarimol, to mention a few, is therefore desirable.

Although GC-MS has also been employed, liquid chromatography linked to tandem mass spectrometry (LC-MS/MS) is the technique that is most frequently used for pesticide detection in beer. Without requiring any conversion procedures, Nagatomi et al. (2013) created an LC-MS/MS approach to concurrently assess beer for glyphosate, glufosinate, and its metabolic metabolites. Commercial canned beer sample analyses were conducted using this technique. The LOQ of 10g kg-1 was assessed to be a suitably low level, despite the fact that residues of glyphosate were discovered in four of the samples. Inoue et al. (2011) followed the fate of pesticides during the brewing process using LC-MS/MS. For this, samples of ground malt were experimentally contaminated with a range of pesticides, and the residual ratios in unhopped wort, spent grain, chilled wort, and the final beer were then examined.

The majority of the pesticides had their content decreased after mashing, and just a few pesticides were still present in the beer in high concentrations. The following pesticides should be used with extra caution on brewing grains and hops: methamidophos, 2-(1-naphthyl) acetamide, imazaquin, fluroxypyr, flumetsulam, thiamethoxam, imibenconazole-desbenzyl, imidacloprid, and tebuthiuron.

8.7 REFERENCES

Alves, V., Gonçalves, J., Figueira, J. A., Ornelas, L. P., Branco, R. N., Câmara, J. S., & Pereira, J. A. (2020). Beer volatile fingerprinting at different brewing steps. *Food Chemistry, 326*, 126856.

Aron, P. M., & Shellhammer, T. H. (2010). A discussion of polyphenols in beer physical and flavour stability. *Journal of the Institute of Brewing, 116*(4), 369–380.

Basalekou, M., Kyraleou, M., & Kallithraka, S. (2022). Authentication of wine and other alcohol-based beverages—future global scenario. In *Future foods* (pp. 669–695). Academic Press.

Bauer, J. I., Gross, M., Gottschalk, C., & Usleber, E. (2016). Investigations on the occurrence of mycotoxins in beer. *Food Control, 63*, 135–139.

Bravi, E., Marconi, O., Sileoni, V., & Perretti, G. (2017). Determination of free fatty acids in beer. *Food Chemistry, 215*, 341–346.

Bryła, M., Ksieniewicz-Wozniak, E., Waskiewicz, A., Szymczyk, K., & Jędrzejczak, R. (2018). Co-occurrence of nivalenol, deoxynivalenol and deoxynivalenol-3-glucoside in beer samples. *Food Control, 92*, 319–324.

Cajka, T., Riddellova, K., Tomaniova, M., & Hajslova, J. (2010). Recognition of beer brand based on multivariate analysis of volatile fingerprint. *Journal of Chromatography A, 1217*(25), 4195–4203.

Castellari, M., Sartini, E., Spinabelli, U., Riponi, C., & Galassi, S. (2001). Determination of carboxylic acids, carbohydrates, glycerol, ethanol, and 5-HMF in beer by high-performance liquid chromatography and UV-refractive index double detection. *Journal of Chromatographic Science, 39*(6), 235–238.

Charry-Parra, G., DeJesus-Echevarria, M., & Perez, F. J. (2011). Beer volatile analysis: Optimization of HS/SPME coupled to GC/MS/FID. *Journal of Food Science, 76*(2), C205–C211.

Fangel, J. U., Eiken, J., Sierksma, A., Schols, H. A., Willats, W. G., & Harholt, J. (2018). Tracking polysaccharides through the brewing process. *Carbohydrate Polymers, 196*, 465–473.

Gorjanovic, S. Z., Novakovic, M. M., Potkonjak, N. I., Leskosek-Cukalovic, I., & Suznjevic, D. Z. (2010). Application of a novel antioxidative assay in beer analysis and brewing process monitoring. *Journal of Agricultural and Food Chemistry, 58*(2), 744–751.

Granato, D., Branco, G. F., Faria, J. D. A. F., & Cruz, A. G. (2011). Characterization of Brazilian lager and brown ale beers based on color, phenolic compounds, and antioxidant activity using chemometrics. *Journal of the Science of Food and Agriculture, 91*(3), 563–571.

He, G., Du, J., Zhang, K., Wei, G., & Wang, W. (2012). Antioxidant capability and potableness of fresh cloudy wheat beer stored at different temperatures. *Journal of the Institute of Brewing, 118*(4), 386–392.

Hernandes, K. C., Souza-Silva, É. A., Assumpção, C. F., Zini, C. A., & Welke, J. E. (2019). Validation of an analytical method using HS-SPME-GC/MS-SIM to assess the exposure risk to carbonyl compounds and furan derivatives through beer consumption. *Food Additives & Contaminants: Part A, 36*(12), 1808–1821.

Inoue, T., Nagatomi, Y., Suga, K., Uyama, A., & Mochizuki, N. (2011). Fate of pesticides during beer brewing. *Journal of Agricultural and Food Chemistry, 59*(8), 3857–3868.

Jiao, C., Zhang, Y., Li, S., & Chen, X. (2021). Flame retardant effect of 1-aminoethyl-3-methylimidazolium hexafluorophosphate in thermoplastic polyurethane elastomer. *Journal of Thermal Analysis and Calorimetry, 145*(1), 173–184.

Krogerus, K., & Gibson, B. R. (2013). 125th anniversary review: Diacetyl and its control during brewery fermentation. *Journal of the Institute of Brewing, 119*(3), 86–97.

Lay, J. O. (2000). MALDI-TOF mass spectrometry and bacterial taxonomy. *TrAC: Trends in Analytical Chemistry, 19*(8), 507–516.

Lehtonen, P., & Hurme, R. (1994). Liquid chromatographic determination of sugars in beer by evaporative light scattering detection. *Journal of the Institute of Brewing, 100*(5), 343–346.

Liguori, L., De Francesco, G., Russo, P., Albanese, D., Perretti, G., & Matteo, M. D. (2015). Quality improvement of low alcohol craft beer produced by evaporative pertraction. *Chemical Engineering, 43*.

Marques, D. R., Cassis, M. A., Quelhas, J. O. F., Bertozzi, J., Visentainer, J. V., Oliveira, C. C., & Monteiro, A. R. G. (2017). Characterization of craft beers and their bioactive compounds. *Chemical Engineering Transactions, 57*, 1747–1752.

Montanari, L., Perretti, G., Natella, F., Guidi, A., & Fantozzi, P. (1999). Organic and phenolic acids in beer. *LWT-Food Science and Technology, 32*(8), 535–539.

Moura-Nunes, N., Brito, T. C., da Fonseca, N. D., de Aguiar, P. F., Monteiro, M., Perrone, D., & Torres, A. G. (2016). Phenolic compounds of Brazilian beers from different types and styles and application of chemometrics for modeling antioxidant capacity. *Food Chemistry, 199*, 105–113.

Nagatomi, Y., Yoshioka, T., Yanagisawa, M., Uyama, A., & Mochizuki, N. (2013). Simultaneous LC-MS/MS analysis of glyphosate, glufosinate, and their metabolic products in beer, barley tea, and their ingredients. *Bioscience, Biotechnology, and Biochemistry, 77*(11), 2218–2221.

Nardini, M., & Garaguso, I. (2020). Characterization of bioactive compounds and antioxidant activity of fruit beers. *Food Chemistry, 305*, 125437.

Oroian, M., Damian, C., Leahu, A., & Gherasim, O. (2016). Polyphenol content and antioxidant activity of commercial beers from the Romanian market. *Food and Environment Safety Journal, 12*(4).

Perez-Ruiz, T., Martınez-Lozano, C., Tomas, V., & Martın, J. (2004). High-performance liquid chromatographic separation and quantification of citric, lactic, malic, oxalic and tartaric acids using a post-column photochemical reaction and chemiluminescence detection. *Journal of Chromatography A, 1026*(1–2), 57–64.

Piazzon, A., Forte, M., & Nardini, M. (2010). Characterization of phenolics content and antioxidant activity of different beer types. *Journal of Agricultural and Food Chemistry, 58*(19), 10677–10683.

Plata, M. R., Koch, C., Wechselberger, P., Herwig, C., & Lendl, B. (2013). Determination of carbohydrates present in Saccharomyces cerevisiae using mid-infrared spectroscopy and partial least squares regression. *Analytical and Bioanalytical Chemistry, 405*(25), 8241–8250.

Rakete, S., & Glomb, M. A. (2013). A novel approach for the quantitation of carbohydrates in mash, wort, and beer with RP-HPLC using 1-naphthylamine for precolumn derivatization. *Journal of Agricultural and Food Chemistry, 61*(16), 3828–3833.

Santos, I. C., Smuts, J., Choi, W. S., Kim, Y., Kim, S. B., & Schug, K. A. (2018). Analysis of bacterial FAMEs using gas chromatography–vacuum ultraviolet spectroscopy for the identification and discrimination of bacteria. *Talanta, 182*, 536–543.

Spitaels, F., Wieme, A. D., Janssens, M., Aerts, M., Daniel, H. M., Van Landschoot, A., De Vuyst, L., & Vandamme, P. (2014). The microbial diversity of traditional spontaneously fermented lambic beer. *PLoS One, 9*(4), e95384.

Spreng, S., & Hofmann, T. (2018). Activity-guided identification of in vitro antioxidants in beer. *Journal of Agricultural and Food Chemistry, 66*(3), 720–731.

Steiner, J., Woods, L., & Watson, P. (2012). *Steiner & Woods EU law*. Oxford University Press.

Stewart, G. G., Russell, I., & Anstruther, A. (Eds.). (2017). *Handbook of brewing*. CRC Press.

Strong, G., & England, K. (2015). *Beer judge certification program style guidelines*. BJCP.

Takahashi, M., Kita, Y., Kusaka, K., Mizuno, A., & Goto-Yamamoto, N. (2015). Evaluation of microbial diversity in the pilot-scale beer brewing process by culture-dependent and culture-independent method. *Journal of Applied Microbiology, 118*(2), 454–469.

Tusekwa, T. C. E., Mosha, H. S., Laswai, E. E., & Towo, A. B. (2000). Traditional alcoholic beverages of Tanzania: Production, quality and changes in quality attributes during storage. *International Journal of Food Sciences and Nutrition, 51*(2), 135–143.

Vanderhaegen, B., Neven, H., Verachtert, H., & Derdelinckx, G. (2006). The chemistry of beer aging–a critical review. *Food Chemistry*, *95*(3), 357–381.

Wieme, A. D., Spitaels, F., Aerts, M., De Bruyne, K., Van Landschoot, A., & Vandamme, P. (2014). Identification of beer-spoilage bacteria using matrix-assisted laser desorption/ionization time-of-flight mass spectrometry. *International Journal of Food Microbiology*, *185*, 41–50.

Wunderlich, S., & Back, W. (2009). Overview of manufacturing beer: Ingredients, processes, and quality criteria. In *Beer in health and disease prevention* (pp. 3–16). Academic Press.

Zeng, W., Chen, Y., Cui, H., Wu, F., Zhu, Y., & Fritz, J. S. (2006). Single-column method of ion chromatography for the determination of common cations and some transition metals. *Journal of Chromatography A*, *1118*(1), 68–72.

Zhao, H., Chen, W., Lu, J., & Zhao, M. (2010). Phenolic profiles and antioxidant activities of commercial beers. *Food Chemistry*, *119*(3), 1150–1158.

9 Antioxidants and Polyphenolic Characteristics of Beers

Beer is a natural beverage that contains organic acids and vitamins, proteins, hops, water, and little to no fat and calories. Beers have superior nutritional value compared to other drinking alcohol because of their minerals and vital nutrients, including calcium, magnesium, potassium, and sodium. Malts and other cereals used for brewing contribute to naturally occurring antioxidant substances like polyphenols in beers.

Antioxidants are substances that are present at low concentrations compared to those of an oxidizable substrate, which significantly slow down or stop that substrate from oxidizing. They act in various ways including complexing redox-catalytic metal ions, scavenging free radicals, and breaking down peroxides. The chemical makeup and concentration of the antioxidant present determine how strong this effect is.

All plant organs contain polyphenolic compounds, which are a crucial component of the human diet. The phenylpropanoid biosynthetic pathway, which also yields a wide range of plant phenols, is responsible for their synthesis. The ability of polyphenolic compounds to bind and precipitate macromolecules (dietary protein, carbohydrate, and digestive enzymes) was the focus of interest in previous decades. However, in the latter half of the 20th century, the antioxidant and free radical–scavenging properties of phenolic compounds in food have drawn more attention.

Beer's growing nutritional appeal is due to its abundance in antioxidant compounds and low ethanol content. Antioxidants are vital substances that protect our health by reducing the oxidative stress brought on by an excess of reactive oxygen or nitrogen species. Reactive oxygen species (ROS) and reactive nitrogen species (RNS) are both collective terms that have been used for a variety of free radicals, including nitric oxide, superoxide, hydroxyl, and peroxyl, as well as for non-radical reactive intermediates like hydrogen peroxide, nitrogen dioxide radicals, and peroxynitrite. Currently, these free radicals are produced by typical physiological processes in our body, but their generation is made worse by pathological circumstances, and they play a significant role in regulatory and pathological processes. They can chelate metal ions, inhibit prooxidative enzymes, and scavenge free radicals in a variety of ways.

9.1 SOURCE OF PHENOLIC COMPOUNDS IN BEER

Antioxidants, phenolic compounds derived from barley and hops that are easily absorbed and extensively metabolized in humans, are found in beer. These antioxidants are highly nutritious and are thought to be potential cancer chemopreventive agents and cardiovascular health promoters. The presence of phenolics in beer has

DOI: 10.1201/b22906-9

technological implications in addition to its physiological function. It is common knowledge that phenolic compounds have an impact on the appearance, flavor, and nonbiological stability of beer. Beer with a high concentration of antioxidants has better, more consistent flavor and aroma as well as foam stability. Additionally, it resists oxidation, which could extend its shelf life. The phenolic content of beer and wine is comparable.

Recent research suggests that red wine and beer have comparable in vivo AO capacity despite having different total polyphenol concentrations. This might be because beer phenolics are easier to absorb than red wine phenolics. Although there are only half as many antioxidants in red wine and twice as many in white wine per drink of equivalent alcohol content, it's possible that the red wine's AOs are larger molecules that are more difficult to absorb than the smaller ones present in beer. The phenolic content of beer, malt, wort, hops, and barley is a topic covered in a wide range of literary works (Gorjanovic et al., 2010).

Antioxidants are the main beer ingredients that contribute to its practical properties. The main naturally occurring antioxidants in beer are polyphenols, which are primarily derived from malt (70–80%) and hops (30%). Simple phenols, aromatic carboxylic acids, and phenol carboxylic acids are among the 78 different phenol compounds that have been identified. Beer type has a significant impact on the antioxidant activity of beer. Dark beers can be compared to rose and white wine, as well as orange juice, but they appear to be significantly inferior to coffee, red wine, and tea.

Hops' cones contain a medicinal component called lupuli strobili. It is a source of the chemical precursors that give beer its distinctively pleasant bitterness and aroma. Aryl phloroglucinols, essential oils, flavonoids, bitter acids, tannins, and resins are all present in them. Hops relax spasms and have a calming and sedative effect. They promote digestion because of their bitter ingredients. Hops polyphenols have significant antioxidant activity.

Malt also plays a role in beer's oxidative stability and is a natural source of antioxidants that can help slow down reactions brought on by ROS. Malt naturally contains antioxidants that can scavenge oxygen-free radicals and inhibit oxidative reactions, preventing the need to add exogenous antioxidant compounds to keep beer's oxidative stability (Vanderhaegen et al., 2006). Malt antioxidants may also significantly improve a consumer's health by preventing and reducing ROS, which are known to be linked to a number of diseases (Landete, 2013).

Lu et al. (2007), Inns et al. (2011), Dvorakova et al. (2008), Leitao et al. (2012), and Samaras et al. (2005) have shown that the malting process and roasting are responsible for changes in the composition of barley and malt grains involving modifications and degradation of endogenous phenolic compounds (Leitao et al., 2012) and the generation of Maillard reaction products (Yahya et al., 2014), with a great impact on the overall antioxidant capacity of malt. In fact, the development of these Maillard products during thermal processing has been associated with a pro-oxidative effect and with a negative effect on the oxidative stability of malt (Carvalho et al., 2016) and beer (Kunz et al., 2013).

The mechanisms behind anti/prooxidant effects of Maillard products are still unclear since their structures are unknown. The mechanisms are assumed to be based on their ability to trap positively charged electrophilic species, to scavenge oxygen radicals, to have reducing power, and to chelate metals to form inactive complexes (Echavarría et al., 2012).

Craft beers differ from commercial beers in that they only use malt and hops as their primary ingredients, are not filtered, and do not contain any additives. While phenolic compounds in beer serve as significant antioxidants with mechanisms for the removal of free radicals, they also interact with proteins during beer storage to produce turbidity. Polyvinylpyrrolidone is used in the clarification process for large-scale brewing, which involves removing phenolic compounds (Marques et al., 2017).

Antioxidant activity has a significant impact on beer quality, and measuring it is essential for both market sales and brewing process optimization. Several assays have been used over the past few years to investigate it.

The majority of breweries are very concerned about shelf-life issues due to the increasing export and consumption of beer. Understanding the processes that cause these changes in aged beer is crucial because the phenomenon of beer ageing is complex.

The biochemical reactions that occur upon storage of beers are at varying rates and also depends on storage conditions. Beers have reducing sugars and other substances that exhibit antioxidants properties, Maillard vitamins, reaction by-products, and phenolic compounds. Polyphenols are important antioxidants with both molecular and cellular mechanisms, free radical scavenging, and metal chelation.

During storage, phenolic compounds in a beer react with proteins to create hazes and high-molecular-weight species (Vanderhaegen et al., 2006). Additionally, it is believed that polyphenols have a minimal impact on the oxidative stability of beer (Andersen et al., 2000). The stability of its finished products is a concern for the brewing industry. Beer loses quality as it is stored, and haze, browning, and the development of unfavorable flavors all take place.

9.2 PHENOLIC COMPOUNDS IN BEER

A group of chemical substances known as phenolic compounds are those that contain at least one phenol unit. According to studies, phenols account for more than half of the antioxidant activity of beer. On the basis of structure, different types of phenols are categorized as phenolic acids, flavonoids, stilbenes, coumarins, lignans, tannins, and chalcones, anthocyanidins, isoflavonoids, flavonols, flavones, and flavanones. The electronic configuration of the phenols allows easy release of electrons to free radical species. This release transfers the radical character to phenol, a radical that is generally more stable than the initial radical species.

The reaction products of phenolic compounds with free radicals are reduced radical species and a phenolic radical. It has been noted that homologous cinnamic acids exhibit a higher antioxidant potential than the respective benzoic acid derivatives and that the antioxidant activity of phenolic acids depends on their chemical structure, particularly on ring substituents. The number of OH substituents in phenols affects their antioxidant activity, and Zhang et al. (2017) observed that the degree of polymerization in proanthocyanidins affects their antioxidant activity. About 70–80% of phenolic compounds come from barley, while 30–20% come from hops.

The addition of hops, cereals, and malt during production increases the amount of naturally occurring antioxidants in beer, particularly phenolic compounds and Maillard reaction sulfites, and reaction by-products (Zhao et al., 2013). Beer contains a variety of polyphenols, including simple phenols, derivatives of benzoic and cinnamic acids, coumarins, catechins, prenylated chalcones, di- and tri-oligomeric proanthocyanidins and iso-α-acids. It's important to point out that phenolic compounds are connected to beer chemicals and affect beer flavor, enhancement of stability, and shelf life (Vanderhaegen et al., 2006), in light of the interest in the impact on beer's stability and sensory quality in comparing the levels of phenolic compounds in various types of beer.

Beer's phenolic content has been quantified to be slightly higher than that of white wine and slightly lower than that of red wine. The varying quality of the raw materials, yeast strains, and brewing process parameters are to blame for this inconsistency.

In barley, phenolic compounds like benzoic and cinnamic acid derivatives, proanthocyanidins, quinines, flavonols, chalcones, flavones, flavanones, and amino phenolic compounds are frequently found in free, esterified, or bound forms. The phenolic acids found in barley grains are ferulic and p-coumaric acid. They can be found in the testa, aleurone, pericarp, husk, and even the endosperm matrix. Vanillic, sinapinic, and p-hydroxybenzoic acids are examples of phenolic acids. Flavan-3-ols derived from monomers ((+)-catechin and ()-epicatechin), dimers (prodelphinidin B3 and procyanidin B3), and trimers (procyanidin C2) are also frequently found in barley.

Beer contains three prenylflavonoids: xanthohumol (XH), isoxanthohumol (IX), and 8-prenylnaringenin (8-PN). They are almost entirely found in hops, which is practically the only food that contains them. Several studies demonstrated that XH exhibits cancer-chemopreventive activities and antimutagenic and anti-carcinogenic properties with an exceptionally broad spectrum of inhibitory mechanisms at all three stages of carcinogenesis: initiation, promotion, and progression. Because it is the strongest phytoestrogen found in nature, 8-PN is of particular interest.

The most significant phenolic compounds found in beer are flavan-3-ol derivatives (catechin, epicatechin, procyanidin, and prodelphinidin), phenolic acids (ferulic, cinnamic, chlorogenic, vanillic, gallic, caffeic, and syringic), and flavonol glycosides. Some phenolic compounds may be eliminated through fining, filtration, or oxidation during the mashing and boiling stages. Additionally, fermentation, maturation, bottling, and storage can result in the reduction or degradation of phenolic components.

Additionally, due to the interaction of polyphenols, proteins, and polysaccharides during beer storage, colloidal haze may develop. By using fining agents like carrageenan, silica gel, or polyvinylpolypyrrolidone, clarification processes can reduce the detrimental effect that malt and hop polyphenols have on the colloidal stability of beer. Nevertheless, these clarification techniques might also lessen the bioactive substances and possible antioxidant activity of the beer.

9.3 PRENYLFLAVONOIDS

A class of flavonoids known as prenylflavonoids are those that have at least one prenyl or geranyl substituent in the ring. The majority of the flavonoids in hops are thought to be precursors to desmethylxanthohumol. Hops also contain other significant prenylflavonoids, including isoxanthohumol, an isomer of xanthohumol, and the two strongest phytoestrogens known to man, 8-prenylnaringenin and 6-prenylnaringenin. A well-known substance is xanthohumol. Although it has been investigated as an anticancer agent, it also exhibits a number of favorable characteristics against pathogenic fungi, malaria, and HIV-1 viruses. It has chemopreventive, sedative, anti-inflammatory, and antimicrobial properties. Even though the isomer of xanthohumol—isoxanthohumol—has proven to be a bit less potent than xanthohumol, it, too, has anti-mutagenic and anti-angiogenic activity. Another chemical compound with anti-carcinogenic properties belonging to this group is 8-prenylnaringenin.

9.4 CATECHINS

The third most prevalent substance in hop cones, flavanol (+)-catechin, has antioxidative and vasodilatory properties. Hops also contain flavanol (-)-epicatechin and (+)-gallocatechin. Catechin and epicatechin, two flavonoids, exhibit anti-inflammatory and antioxidant properties. Compared to individual flavanols and proanthocyanidins, a mixture of hop proanthocyanidins exhibits stronger antioxidant effects.

9.5 FLAVONOLS

The antioxidant flavanols found in fruits, vegetables, hops, and other foods that receive the most attention are quercetin and kaempferol. The most prevalent form of quercetin in hops is rutin, which is the least bioavailable form of quercetin. Plants typically contain flavonols in the form of glycosides, which, in the case of quercetin, presents its bioavailable form. It is well known for having anti-ageing benefits. Various cancer cells can grow more slowly when quercetin and kaempferol are present.

9.6 MULTIFIDOL AND MULTIFIDOL GLUCOSIDES

The following compounds are found in hops: 1-(2-methyl propanoyl)phloroglucinol-glucopyranoside, multifidol glucosides, 1-(3-methyl butyryl) phloroglucinol, and 5-(2 methylpropanoyl) phloroglucinol. The lowest concentration was found for co-multifidol glucopyranoside, demonstrating that minor hop compounds may act as significant taste carriers.

Hops' ferulic acid is classified as a highly antioxidative polyphenolic compound that inhibits lipid peroxidation, shields healthy cells from apoptosis, and neutralizes free radicals. It is crucial for the brewing industry because it slows down iso-acid deterioration and actively guards against beer spoilage. Numerous characteristics of ferulic acid increase the toxicity of some chemicals, carcinogens, and ionizing radiation. It effectively absorbs UV light. It may, however, function as an anti-inflammatory, anti-apoptotic, and anti-carcinogenic agent when combined with specific enzymes. According to some reports, resveratrol has anti-inflammatory and anti-cancer properties and prevents the development of cardiovascular diseases. It is also recognized as an anti-ageing agent by the cosmetics industry.

Endogenous phenolic compounds are degraded as a result of the malting process, which alters the composition of the barley grain. According to a number of authors, malt may contain more phenolic compounds than barley. The fact that the major groups, however, are unchanged suggests that malt has a more pronounced extraction of flavonoids and phenolic acids. Following malting and brewing, polyphenol behavior is discussed in the sections that follow.

The differences in raw materials, the brewing process, and the original gravity all affect a beer's phenolic acid profile. Beer polyphenols can be identified qualitatively (presence or absence), quantitatively, and so-called relative quantitatively fingerprint. The current trend is to analyze each compound separately for detection and quantification because the methods for analyzing total phenol content are not specific for phenolic compounds because they can interact with other reducing substances.

High-performance liquid chromatography (HPLC) is most frequently used for identifying phenolic compounds because of its high sensitivity and selectivity. Up to 47 phenolic compounds have been quantified using more sophisticated and intricate techniques, such as liquid chromatography in combination with an electrospray ionization hybrid linear ion trap quadrupole mass spectrometer (LC-ESI-LQT-Orbitrap-MS).

The concentration of the samples is a crucial and essential step because the individual determination of the phenols present in beer is typically complicated because these compounds are typically found in low concentrations. One option is to use HPLC after a preliminary stage of separation using cartridges. This method allows for the measurement of flavonols and phenolic acids derived from benzoic and cinnamic acids. This methodology was used in later studies with samples of traditional beers. It is significant to note that Martinez et al. (2019) used a single preparation stage to conduct simultaneous determination of nitrogen compounds and phenolic compounds. Acidifying the samples in order to carry out a liquid-liquid extraction followed by HPLC is an alternative to using cartridges.

Beer contains more than 50 phenolic compounds that have been identified. Martinez et al. (2019) observed 12 new phenolic compounds in beers for the first time; the study of phenolic compounds in beer is continuously providing phenolic compounds that had never been identified before. Ferulic, gallic, and p-coumaric acids are generally considered to be the most prevalent phenolic compounds in beer, although vanillic and synaptic acids have also been mentioned as significant phenolic acids in this alcoholic beverage. While gallic acid predominates in Brazilian and Serbian beers, ferulic acid is the most prevalent phenolic acid in Chinese, Chilean, and European beers.

According to the type of beer, the most prevalent acid in ales is caffeic acid, while gallic acid is more prevalent in lagers. In non-alcoholic black, abbey, wheat, Pilsen, and bock beers, ferulic acid predominates. Due to its positive effects on health, xanthohumol, which can be found in concentrations between 0.002 mg/L and 0.628 mg/L, is one of the most significant antioxidants. Beer contains more of this compound due to roasted malts. Lager and alcohol-free beers contain less resveratrol, another polyphenol of great interest, than ale-type beers.

9.7 MELANOIDINS

Maillard reactions, which take place during the malting and brewing processes, produce melanoidins, which are macromolecular, nitrogenous, and brown in color.

The first step involves the condensation of a free amino group found in peptides or proteins with a carbonyl group, typically from a reducing sugar. An Amadori rearrangement product is produced as a result, and it can react further to produce colored low-molecular-mass products and melanoidins. The time and temperature used during the brewing process affect the Maillard reaction products. High-reactive intermediates are polymerized to create high-molecular-weight (HMW) compounds in the Maillard reaction's later stages.

The polymerization of early-formed low-molecular-weight (LMW) compounds (10 kDa) into HMW brown compounds (> 300 kDa) is caused by malt roasting, which is why roasted malts have less LMW than pale malts. As a result, roasted malts are distinguished by intense brown HMW colorants while pale and caramel malts are distinguished by light brown LMW colorants. The physiological relevance of melanoidin's biological activities is constrained by two main factors. It is difficult to pinpoint the active principles in charge of a given biological activity due to our limited understanding of the structure of food melanoidins. Second, despite being a common component of the average person's diet, melanoidins are typically regarded as poorly bioavailable and poorly absorbable substances. Food melanoidin's structural characteristics are largely unknown. It is assumed that it lacks a clear structure and that its composition and the molar concentration of the parent reacting compounds, as well as the reaction's temperature, pH, and heating time, all play a significant role. Because of their diversity and heterogeneity, food melanoidins are notoriously difficult to study structurally.

9.8 MELANOIDIN CONTENT MEASUREMENTS

The quantitative analysis of melanoidins has drawbacks, and the typical method of accounting for melanoid content entails three steps: first, an extraction is carried out, and then comes an ultracentrifugation, and finally, the solution is lyophilized. The yellow extract obtained yields the total amount of melanoidin.

Dark blond alcohol-free beers have the highest melanoidin content, per published studies. This content varies depending on the raw material and the specific brewing process, ranging from 0.58 mg/L for alcohol-free beer to 0.61 mg/L for blond beer to 1.49 mg/L for dark beers (Martinez et al., 2019).

Since black beers are made from more roasted malt than blond beers, they typically contain more melanoidin than blond beers do. Pale malts typically have less reducing power than more colored malts for the wort and beer. The malt is dried in a kiln for up to 30 hours, producing a stable end product that is simple to handle, store, and mill. The higher temperatures required to produce color compounds like melanoidin and phenolic species are linked to the reducing power. Higher levels of antioxidants (reductones and melanoidins) are formed during MR as a result of the higher temperatures used to create special dark malts. Dark malt beers typically have a longer shelf life than pale beers because of this (Martinez et al., 2019).

The study by Hellwig et al. (2016) on the Maillard reaction products (MRPs) found in beer is an intriguing one. They measured seven MRPs using HPLC-ESI-MS/MS in the multiple reaction monitoring modes in various types of beer, including pilsner, dark, bock, wheat, and non-alcoholic beverages using the conventional addition procedure. There was a high-molecular-weight component. Prior to analysis, the substance was dialysis isolated and enzymatically hydrolyzed. The findings showed that Fructosyl lysine (6.8–27.0 mg/L) and maltulosyllysine (3.7–21.8 mg/L) are significant free MRPs in beer. Additionally, the analyzed beers had relatively high concentrations of late-stage free MRPs like mg-H1 (0.3–2.5 mg/L), pyrraline (0.2–1.6 mg/L), formyline in trace amounts (4–230 µg/L), argpyrimidine (0.1–4.1 µg/L), and maltosine (6–56 µg/L).

Recent studies were successful in isolating a low-molecular-weight yellow pigment from black beer. This pigment, identified as perlolyrine (a by-product of the tryptophan Maillard reaction), was found in various types of beer at a concentration of 3.2–14.0 µg/100 mL. Maillard reaction products can act as antioxidants through a number of different mechanisms, including oxygen scavengers, reactive oxygen scavengers, reducing agents, and metal chelating agents. It has been established that using colored malt increases the finished beer's stability, and it has also been demonstrated that darker beers retain more reducing power when stored. The existence of positive correlations between antioxidant activity and malt color was demonstrated by numerous studies, which have attributed them to the presence of Maillard components. More recently, Zhao et al. (2013) discovered that the antioxidant capacity of beers and their melanoidin content correlated positively.

9.9 TOTAL PHENOLIC CONTENT MEASUREMENT

There are several analytical methods for determining the total phenol content (TPC) in beers, most of which are based on the reaction of the phenols with a colorimetric reagent and the measurement of the colored product's absorption in the visible region of the spectrum. Total phenol content (TPC) is typically expressed as gallic acid equivalents (GAE). These assays exhibit extremely variable specificity, and it is frequently necessary to consider the contribution of additional compound groups.

The Bishop's method, the Prussian blue assay, and the Folin-Ciocalteu method (FC) are the three best-known traditional techniques for measuring total phenol content. The FC reagent, which is a mixture of phosphomolybdate and phosphotungstate, is reduced by polyphenols using the Folin-Ciocalteu method, and absorption measured at 260 nm. Under alkaline conditions, the reduction reaction is accelerated since the Folin-Ciocalteu reaction's basis for color formation is the reagent's chemical reduction. Bishop's method, which the European Brewery Convention (EBC) has approved as an official method, is a second approach for calculating the TPC (EBC method 9.11). The sample is mixed with carboxymethyl cellulose/ethylenediaminetetraacetic acid reagent (CMC/EDTA), and CMC is then added to improve transparency while EDTA is used as an antiseptic. This spectrophotometric method is based on a chelation reaction between the polyphenols and Fe(III) in basic medium. The absorbance at 600 nm is then measured after that. Results from the Bishop assay typically show lower polyphenol concentrations than those from the FC assay because they are more selective.

Because non-phenolic compounds rarely interfere with the Prussian blue assay, it is an effective method for determining phenols. This method is based on the reduction of ferricyanide ions $[Fe(CN)_6]^{3-}$ to ferrocyanide ions $[Fe(CN)_6]^{4-}$ by the reaction of phenols with the latter. Prussian blue, also known as ferric ferrocyanide $Fe_4[Fe(CN)_6]^3$, is created when an excess of iron (III) reacts with a ferrocyanide ion, and its absorbance at 700 nm is measured.

The majority of current techniques for calculating the TPC rely on combining the use of enzymes and electroanalytical methods. On the basis of enzymes like tyrosinase, laccase, and peroxidase, biosensors for polyphenol detection have been developed using various electrode materials, flow systems, and sample pretreatment techniques with shorter analysis times. Phenols are enzymatically oxidized to quinones or radicals, and then their reduction currents are used to detect them at the electrode. Wineries are particularly interested in these techniques because they have several advantages over conventional techniques, including straightforward instrumentation, sensitivity, quick response, no sample treatment, low cost, compact size, and the potential for in situ and online analysis. Additionally, it has been observed that there are no appreciable differences between the outcomes produced by these methods and those produced by the FC method.

It is well known that different types of beer have different profiles of total polyphenols and phenolic acids. The highest TPC values are typically found in fruity and dark beers, while the lowest TPC values are found in alcohol-free brews. Beers like bock, abbey, ale, and lager fall somewhere in the middle. Numerous studies show fruits are a significant source of phenols, and fruity beers have high phenolic content. For a Belgian beer, values of 1033 mg GAE/L have been attained using the FC method. Also, highest values of TPC were observed in persimmon- or banana-based beers or goji berries.

Dark beers are positioned second in terms of phenolic content. According to published studies, this type of beer should contain at least 300 mg GAE/L of phenol and up to 943 mg GAE/L of phenol, which was the value discovered by Granato et al. (2011) for a beer aged with sour cherry. Granato et al. (2011) compared additional dark beers to pale beers and found similar results to those found previously, with higher values for dark beers (280–525 vs 119–200 mg GAE/L). Due to the higher proportion of malted barley and the production of polyphenols during the malting process, dark beers have higher TPC.

The lowest values for TPC are found in alcohol-free beers. Alcohol-free beers are usually brewed with less original wort extract and inhibition of alcohol formation or as normal alcoholic beers with alcohol removal at the last step. The fact that alcohol-free beers present a lower TPC is important because it indicates that the beer was not developed with techniques that remove alcohol without altering the remaining compounds (phenols); such techniques can be dealcoholization of beer by reverse osmosis or the use of membranes. TPC for alcohol-free beer varies between 75 and 366 mg GAE/L.

Beers without alcohol have the lowest TPC values. Beers that are alcohol-free are typically brewed with less original wort extract and alcohol formation inhibition or as regular alcoholic beers with the alcohol removed at the very end. The fact that alcohol-free beers have a lower TPC is significant because it shows that these beers were not created using methods that dealcoholize beer using reverse osmosis or membranes without changing the remaining compounds (phenols). TPC for beer without alcohol ranges from 75 to 366 mg GAE/L. The majority of research focuses on figuring out how much phenols are in lager beers. In this regard, Zhao et al. (2010) conducted a thorough study that included the analysis of 34 lager beers with TPC ranging from 152 to 339 mg GAE/L.

9.10 METHODS OF ANTIOXIDANT MEASUREMENT

The methods for calculating the level of activity in wort and beer have been reviewed by Karabin. Studies on the effectiveness of barley, malt, and hops in antioxidants are also reported. Studies have been conducted to determine how the malting, mashing, and brewing processes affect the hue, flavor, concentration of phenolic compounds, and antioxidant potential of malt, wort, and beer. In general, commonly used assays are time consuming and frequently require reactive species.

The reducing power is frequently linked to antioxidant activity and may be an important sign of this activity. Certain substances exhibit antioxidant activity by chelating metal ions. Reactive oxygen species that take part in the oxidation of beer and produce unpleasant flavors can be created by metal ions like iron or copper. The methods to assess antioxidant capacity are divided into two broad categories based on the reaction mechanisms used in the processes that reduce free radicals: methods based on single electron transfer (SET) and methods based on hydrogen atom transfer (HAT).

In SET methods, the antioxidant gives the free radical an electron, and the antioxidant then changes into a radical cation. In the second method, the antioxidant loses one hydrogen atom to the free radical, and the antioxidant then changes into a radical. The HAT and SET processes that phenolic compounds can go through largely depend on their chemical makeup. The substances most likely to refer to HAT are tocopherol, hydroxytyrosol, gallic acid, caffeic acid, and epicatechin. For SET, resveratrol and kaempferol work better. It can be assumed that HAT is the antioxidant mechanism that occurs most frequently in beer since several studies have shown that gallic acid and caffeic acid are the main phenols present in beer.

According to Gerhauser (2005), hops (*Humulus lupulus* L.) contain α-acids (humulones), β-acids (lupulones), and polyphenols like prenylated flavonoids. A sizable number of phenolic compounds, such as hydroxycinnamic acids (e.g., p-coumaric, ferulic, chlorogenic, and caffeic acids) and phenolic acids, are found in monomeric form (e.g., gallic acid). Ferulic acid is the most significant hydroxycinnamic acid derived from barley.

In terms of its antioxidant properties, xanthohumol is regarded as the most significant polyphenol because it exhibits the highest total oxygen radical absorbance capacity and the highest singlet oxygen absorbance capacity (Yamaguchi et al., 2009). It has been recognized as a broad-spectrum cancer chemopreventive agent with inhibitory effects on carcinogenesis's initiation, promotion, and progression stages (Gerhauser, 2005). It is important to note that xanthohumol is a prenylated chalcone with a straightforward structural makeup that only appears in hop plants. As a result, research interest and investigation are focused on the hops-containing beers, which are thought to be the primary dietary source of the related prenylflavonoids (Stevens & Page, 2004).

Polak et al. (2013) used electron paramagnetic resonance (EPR) spectroscopy to examine the antioxidant qualities of various types of beers. They reported that the value of the antioxidant capacity significantly (0.05 level of significance) depends on the amount of extract and the color of the beer, according to an analysis of variance. Although the antioxidant qualities of beer are not affected by the alcohol content or the type of fermentation, it appears that additives do so to some extent. Monitoring the changes in the EPR spectrum's intensity caused by interactions between the antioxidants in a beer sample and the stable radical DPPH allowed for this (1,1-diphenyl-2-picrylhydrazyl).

In Trolox equivalents, such as 1M Trolox in a 100mL sample of beer, the antioxidant capacity was then shown. The type, color, extract content, and alcohol all had an impact on the antioxidant activities of commercial beer samples; this was discovered using two-way hierarchical clustering and analysis of variance. In Trolox equivalents, such as 1M Trolox in a 100mL sample of beer, the antioxidant capacity was then shown. The type, color, extract content, and alcohol all had an impact on the antioxidant activities of commercial beer samples; this was discovered using two-way hierarchical clustering and analysis of variance.

9.11 BIOACTIVITY AND HUMAN METABOLISM

Despite the toxicity of ethanol, beverages make up about 4–6% of the average energy intake in the majority of Western countries. The concentrations of minerals, polyphenols, trace elements, and antioxidants, as well as the nutrients found in malt, hops, and beer in considerable amount. Blood homocysteine levels and certain vitamin concentrations in beer that are crucial health indicators have been examined (Gorinstein et al., 2007).

Some researchers claimed that alcohol has a cardioprotective effect. On the basis of the antioxidant properties of beer polyphenols, moderate alcohol use enhances lipid metabolism and raises antioxidant and anticoagulant activity. Despite the effectiveness of preventive measures, hypercholesterolemia continues to be the primary risk factor for atherosclerosis, which makes it one of the most dangerous diseases in Western industrialized countries.

Only LDL-C particles that have undergone oxidation can pierce the walls of arteries and obstruct them. By preventing the production of superoxide, the polyphenol action could protect the integrity of endothelial function. Additionally, these antioxidants may hinder the oxidation of low-density lipoproteins and control macrophage attack on the endothelium. According to the majority of researchers, monitoring oxidized LDL-C is necessary to identify it as a marker for the prevention of atherosclerosis (Gorinstein et al., 2007). According to some studies (Sierksma et al., 2002), moderate alcohol consumption is associated with a decreased risk of cardiovascular disease.

9.12 REFERENCES

Andersen, M. L., Outtrup, H., & Skibsted, L. H. (2000). Potential antioxidants in beer assessed by ESR spin trapping. *Journal of Agricultural and Food Chemistry*, *48*(8), 3106–3111.

Carvalho, F. R., Wang, Q. J., Van Ee, R., & Spence, C. (2016). The influence of soundscapes on the perception and evaluation of beers. *Food Quality and Preference*, *52*, 32–41.

Dvorakova, M., Guido, L. F., Dostálek, P., Skulilová, Z., Moreira, M. M., & Barros, A. A. (2008). Antioxidant properties of free, soluble ester and insoluble-bound phenolic compounds in different barley varieties and corresponding malts. *Journal of the Institute of Brewing*, *114*(1), 27–33.

Echavarría, A. P., Pagán, J., & Ibarz, A. (2012). Melanoidins formed by Maillard reaction in food and their biological activity. *Food Engineering Reviews*, *4*(4), 203–223.

Gerhauser, B. C., C., Knauft, J., Zapp, J., & Becker, H. (2005). Anti-inflammatory acylphloroglucinol derivatives from hops (*Humulus lupulus*). *Journal of Natural Products*, *68*(10), 1545–1548.

Gorinstein, S., Vargas, O. J. M., Jaramillo, N. O., Salas, I. A., Ayala, A. L. M., Arancibia-Avila, P., & Trakhtenberg, S. (2007). The total polyphenols and the antioxidant potentials of some selected cereals and pseudocereals. *European Food Research and Technology*, *225*(3), 321–328.

Gorjanovic, S. Z., Novakovic, M. M., Potkonjak, N. I., Leskosek-Cukalovic, I., & Suznjevic, D. Z. (2010). Application of a novel antioxidative assay in beer analysis and brewing process monitoring. *Journal of Agricultural and Food Chemistry*, *58*(2), 744–751.

Granato, D., Branco, G. F., Faria, J. D. A. F., & Cruz, A. G. (2011). Characterization of Brazilian lager and brown ale beers based on color, phenolic compounds, and antioxidant activity using chemometrics. *Journal of the Science of Food and Agriculture*, *91*(3), 563–571.

Hellwig, M., Witte, S., & Henle, T. (2016). Free and protein-bound Maillard reaction products in beer: Method development and a survey of different beer types. *Journal of Agricultural and Food Chemistry*, *64*(38), 7234–7243.

Inns, E. L., Buggey, L. A., Booer, C., Nursten, H. E., & Ames, J. M. (2011). Effect of modification of the kilning regimen on levels of free ferulic acid and antioxidant activity in malt. *Journal of Agricultural and Food Chemistry*, *59*(17), 9335–9343.

Kunz, T., Strähmel, A., Cortés, N., Kroh, L. W., & Methner, F. J. (2013). Influence of intermediate Maillard reaction products with enediol structure on the oxidative stability of beverages. *Journal of the American Society of Brewing Chemists*, *71*(3), 114–123.

Landete, J. M. (2013). Dietary intake of natural antioxidants: Vitamins and polyphenols. *Critical Reviews in Food Science and Nutrition*, *53*(7), 706–721.

Leitao, C., Marchioni, E., Bergaentzlé, M., Zhao, M., Didierjean, L., Miesch, L., & Ennahar, S. (2012). Fate of polyphenols and antioxidant activity of barley throughout malting and brewing. *Journal of Cereal Science*, *55*(3), 318–322.

Lu, J., Zhao, H., Chen, J., Fan, W., Dong, J., Kong, W., Sun, J., Cao, Y., & Cai, G. (2007). Evolution of phenolic compounds and antioxidant activity during malting. *Journal of Agricultural and Food Chemistry*, *55*(26), 10994–11001.

Marques, D. R., Cassis, M. A., Quelhas, J. O. F., Bertozzi, J., Visentainer, J. V., Oliveira, C. C., & Monteiro, A. R. G. (2017). Characterization of craft beers and their bioactive compounds. *Chemical Engineering Transactions*, *57*, 1747–1752.

Martinez, P., Kerr, W. C., Subbaraman, M. S., & Roberts, S. C. (2019). New estimates of the mean ethanol content of beer, wine, and spirits sold in the United States show a greater increase in per capita alcohol consumption than previous estimates. *Alcoholism: Clinical and Experimental Research*, *43*(3), 509-521.

Pérez-Jiménez, J., Arranz, S., Tabernero, M., Díaz-Rubio, M. E., Serrano, J., Goñi, I., & Saura-Calixto, F. (2008). Updated methodology to determine antioxidant capacity in plant foods, oils and beverages: Extraction, measurement and expression of results. *Food Research International*, *41*(3), 274–285.

Samaras, T. S., Camburn, P. A., Chandra, S. X., Gordon, M. H., & Ames, J. M. (2005). Antioxidant properties of kilned and roasted malts. *Journal of Agricultural and Food Chemistry*, *53*(20), 8068–8074.

Sierksma, A., Van Der Gaag, M. S., Kluft, C., & Hendriks, H. F. J. (2002). Moderate alcohol consumption reduces plasma C-reactive protein and fibrinogen levels; a randomized, diet-controlled intervention study. *European Journal of Clinical Nutrition*, *56*(11), 1130–1136.

Stevens, J. F., & Page, J. E. (2004). Xanthohumol and related prenylflavonoids from hops and beer: To your good health! *Phytochemistry*, *65*(10), 1317–1330.

Tafulo, P. A. R., Queirós, R. B., Delerue-Matos, C. M., & Sales, M. G. F. (2010). Control and comparison of the antioxidant capacity of beers. *Food Research International*, *43*(6), 1702–1709.

Vanderhaegen, B., Neven, H., Verachtert, H., & Derdelinckx, G. (2006). The chemistry of beer aging–A critical review. *Food Chemistry*, *95*(3), 357–381.

Yahya, H., Linforth, R. S., & Cook, D. J. (2014). Flavour generation during commercial barley and malt roasting operations: A time course study. *Food Chemistry*, *145*, 378–387.

Yamaguchi, N., Satoh-Yamaguchi, K., & Ono, M. (2009). In vitro evaluation of antibacterial, anticollagenase, and antioxidant activities of hop components (*Humulus lupulus*) addressing acne vulgaris. *Phytomedicine*, *16*(4), 369–376.

Zhang, R., Huang, L., Deng, Y., Chi, J., Zhang, Y., Wei, Z., & Zhang, M. (2017). Phenolic content and antioxidant activity of eight representative sweet corn varieties grown in South China. *International journal of food properties*, 20(12), 3043–3055.

Zhao, H., Li, H., Sun, G., Yang, B., & Zhao, M. (2013). Assessment of endogenous antioxidative compounds and antioxidant activities of lager beers. *Journal of the Science of Food and Agriculture, 93(4)*, 910–917.

Zhao, H., Chen, W., Lu, J., & Zhao, M. (2010). Phenolic profiles and antioxidant activities of commercial beers. *Food Chemistry*, *119*(3), 1150–1158.

10 Future Aspects

One of the oldest and most popular drinks in the world is beer. Since beer has been produced for 5,000 years, many people believe that it was the first essential component to the development of a civilized society—even before bread. We are constantly coming up with novel methods to improve the first beverage of civilization thousands of years later.

With the rise in customer desire for diversity in beer and the popularity of craft and microbrewing, there has been a movement against the homogeneous production of beer in recent decades. Craft beer sales increased by 4% in volume in the United States in 2018, whereas overall beer volume sales decreased by 1%. Craft beer output increased by 0.8% among Society of Independent Brewers Association members in the UK. This has led to an increase in the variety of ingredients and a rekindled interest in various yeasts and fermenting bacteria to produce novel tastes for a growing number of discerning consumers (Mellor et al., 2020).

With about 5,000 breweries in the United States alone, the microbrewery boom that started around 2008 was still very much in force 10 years later. For instance, there is a craft brewery on almost every block in Seattle, where there are about 200 breweries operating inside the city boundaries. Craft brewers have pushed their creative limits in an effort to separate from a burgeoning field of rivals. In India, craft microbreweries started in 2008. Now India has more than 500 microbreweries. Craft-brewing culture is expanding day by day. We have so many innovations in brewing, just because of this booming craft beer culture.

10.1 NEW TECHNOLOGIES

When we consider innovation, technology comes to mind right away. As a result, we come across instances of research or initiatives in which technology is the main focus. We can take the manufacture of craft beer as an example, monitoring and managing organoleptic parameters using a computerized system with biosensors. Within 12 hours after being harvested, hops—a volatile ingredient—must be added to the brewing recipe. IoT-enabled sensors can make sure they perform at their best.

Microbreweries have recently pushed for technologies like carbon collecting to be more ecologically friendly and decrease waste. The goal is to decrease CO_2 emissions, lower brewing expenses, and recycle CO_2 that would otherwise be discarded for use in other brewing processes. According to some experts, this might help brewers save tens of thousands of dollars annually.

10.2 NEW YEASTS

Due in major part to consumer demand for a variety of products, the brewing business is now going through a period of upheaval and innovation. Innovation need not,

DOI: 10.1201/b22906-10

however, be technological; there is still opportunity for advancement, for example, in yeasts, which are important to the diverse tastes and fragrances of beer. Fermentation requires the hard-to-control live creature known as yeast. We can use the research on aromagenesis—generation of new yeast strains for improved flavors and aromas in beer and wine—as an illustration. This project will offer scientific innovation as well as brand-new, exciting opportunities for the major fermentation industries and emerging small and medium-sized businesses engaged in craft beer brewing.

For beer enthusiasts, new yeasts represent the most exciting development to date. Although yeast is a crucial component of the brewing process, craft beer producers have become hooked on hops in their pursuit of novel tastes. Currently, yeast is very much on their minds, in terms of both cultivating it in labs and locating novel variants in the wild to test in novel brews.

For the future development of yeast strains relevant to brewing, recent developments in DNA sequencing technology, as well as creative uses of more traditional genetic approaches, offer a lot of promise. "Classic" genetic modification techniques, genome shuffling, controlled production of hybrid yeasts, and more contemporary approaches for less intrusive genetic alterations of genomes are among the techniques used.

Novel yeast strains produced through both intraspecific and interspecific (mating between two strains of the same species) yeast hybridizations have been commercialized in industries like biofuels and wine. It is evident that recent findings from whole-genome sequencing, along with advancements in genetic techniques, make it easier and possibly more rewarding than ever to conduct imaginative hybridizations using brewing yeasts. For instance, in the wine industry, interspecific hybrids between numerous different *Saccharomyces* genus members have been created via the rare mating method, using a diploid wine yeast as the *S. cerevisiae* parent; the hybrids frequently produce distinctive and appealing sensory characteristics in wine, and some of the strains are now being used commercially (Bellon et al., 2011, 2013, 2015).

There is a trend in favor of this research in the beer industry as novel lager-like yeast hybrids are starting to be purposefully created in order to create strains with distinctive fermentation, flavor, and aroma characteristics. This is due to the recent discovery of free-living *S. eubayanus* as the non-*S. cerevisiae* component of the lager yeast genome (Mertens et al., 2015). Research on de novo *S. cerevisiae* and *S. eubayanus* hybrids for low-temperature lager brewing has been sparked by the discovery of the psychrotolerant *S. eubayanus*, which has also sparked renewed interest in the functional significance of hybrid organisms and the mechanisms that determine hybrid genome function and stability.

The variety of aroma profiles and other features present in ale yeasts, including "heirloom" strains (Parker et al., 2015), have been emphasized through phenotypic screens (Steensels et al., 2014). The variety of different ale yeasts that can act as the *S. cerevisiae* parent, along with the relatively recent isolation of several genetically diverse and geographically remote strains of *S. eubayanus* point to an expanding universe of potential "lager-like" hybrid combinations (Bing et al., 2014; Peris et al., 2014; Baker et al., 2015). It seems that deliberate intraspecific hybridization has received less attention from researchers studying brewing strains than interspecific hybridization, for example, when it comes to crossing different strains of *S. cerevisiae* yeast. This may be due to the fact that lager beer is by far the most popular type of beer in the world, making it more likely that research to improve lager yeasts will take place and/or be financially feasible.

In general, experimental hybridization research may enhance genetic variety that may then be screened/selected for innovative and desirable characteristics in a brewing environment, which has not been fully investigated. Additionally, intergeneric yeast hybrids, which are primarily created through protoplast fusion, have been investigated in other industrial applications but not in brewing yeasts (Morales & Dujon, 2012; Steensels & Verstrepen, 2014); this method may offer a variety of strains with even more interesting traits.

Genome shuffles are used to combine features or to find the genetic underpinnings of phenotypic qualities in brewing yeasts. Other genetic methods that combine and/or mix the genomes of different strains provide additional options for creating brewing yeast strains. It is impossible to simply marry two non-mating brewing strains to combine their genomes (as one can do with stably haploid, HO-mutant laboratory strains) since almost all of them are aneuploid, diploid, or greater ploidy strains. To quickly combine desirable features from two or more brewing yeast strains into a single strain, it is sometimes possible to undertake mass spore mating or mass cell fusion. These methods can also be used to initiate diverse strains, such as mixed populations (for example, a mutagenized population of cells or a pool of meiotically recombined cells). First, a very large number of cells (or spores, if the strains can produce viable spores) are produced from each initial "parental" population (note that there can be one, two, or even more initial populations); they are then all mixed together, allowing random mating to take place (with haploid cells or spores) or random cell fusion to happen (if asexual cells are converted into protoplasts).

As a result, the genotypes of the several starting populations are mixed into a single cell, frequently producing cells with the combined features of interest. Multiple rounds of mass mating (or mass fusion) followed by selection can be carried out iteratively to further refine or strengthen the expression of the desired phenotypic features if selection or enrichment for cells containing the appropriate mix of traits is achievable. Under the terms of evolution, this process entails genetic recombination, followed by the natural selection over multiple generations of genotypes exhibiting beneficial phenotypes in the enforced environmental state.

A stable hybrid line that displays the required features has often been the aim of these common mass-mating or mass-fusion techniques. The genetic underpinnings of phenotypic features critical to the production of beer may be discovered using related procedures that result in "genome shuffling," and these techniques may also be useful for creating new strains that combine advantageous qualities.

Genome-shuffling experiments are similar to mass-mating or mass-fusion methods, but they are carried out in a way that ensures genome recombination takes place after every round, eventually mixing the two starting genomes together into single cells, but in a very patchwork manner that differs from cell to cell, allowing different phenotypic combinations to be observed. Once more, this may be utilized to combine and improve several beneficial features from various origins into one superior strain. The sites of the genes influencing the phenotypes can also be mapped using the recombined populations.

In particular, genome research has shed light on the steps that led to the domestication of brewing yeast and discovered domestication signals that might be used to further yeast development. In order to produce flavorful non-alcoholic beers as well as novel flavors for existing beers, the functional qualities of non-traditional yeast (both *Saccharomyces* and non-*Saccharomyces*) are being evaluated (Gibson et al., 2017).

Overall, brewing yeasts may be genetically modified using a wide range of methods to change or improve a variety of traits, from fermentation behavior to sensory profile. The brewing industry is anticipated to be significantly and directly impacted by the increased diversity of yeast that can be used in brewing as well as a better understanding of the evolutionary history and biology of yeasts, with potential for increased brewing efficiency, product diversity, and, most importantly, customer satisfaction.

10.3 BARLEY VARIETIES

Utilizing "conventional plant breeding" techniques, barley lines are enhanced by producing crosses through the regular pollination process, which results in the mixing of thousands of genes from the male and female halves of the cross. The ability of the breeder to now know so much more about which genes are dispersed in which breeding lines and how those genes relate to the yield, quality, and weather adaptability attributes the breeder is concurrently seeking to enhance is what has changed in modern plant breeding. The tremendous investment in biotechnology for the medical and industrial sectors has led to an increase in the sophistication and affordability of the instruments used to investigate genetics. The barley industry is turning out to be an encouraging example of how a new business model has emerged that could not only help barley with its triple challenge, but could also allow many more crops to have necessary, advanced tools for breeding goals. For a time, only the largest crops with the largest seed company players could really afford to keep up with the state-of-the-art, data-enabled version of "traditional breeding."

A start-up in St. Louis by the name of Benson Hill has created a data and analytics platform it refers to as CropOS, which stands for crop "operating system." It has a substantial amount of information that is readily accessible regarding the genetics and performance of barley that has been produced by a wide range of governmental and private barley breeding initiatives throughout the world. Breeders may now receive far better advice on how to generate the most productive crosses because of the combination of all of that data and the quality screening procedure that was applied to it. They may then concentrate their crucial local evaluation efforts, which provide new data to the model.

Good new barley lines have historically taken between 9 and 12 years to develop. It could be feasible to reduce that time by half with the CropOS tool. About 80% of potential field evaluations may be avoided by having as much information as possible about which prospective crosses will combine the proper genes, allowing the resources to be concentrated on only the most promising combinations.

The system's major feature, according to Benson Hill, is that it serves as an example of a cooperative community model. CropOS gathers information from both public and private sources, enabling innovators to find and create traits more quickly. The value of their shared data is greater for all parties.

Anheuser-Busch (AB) collaborates with various breeding organizations in addition to its own efforts to grow barley. To improve the CropOS platform, they have provided some of their genetics and performance data.

Because the brewer must provide guidelines on the kinds it wants to be cultivated in each location to achieve its quality criteria, the majority of barley is farmed under contract. A buyer like AB is more likely to be able to suggest excellent alternatives for their contracted producers in the shared breeding data model and to see those good options evolve over time as needed. Additionally, AB has a community outreach program called Smart Barley that aids farmers in selecting the best options for growing these premium types. The agronomic aspects and how they combine with other sustainability and soil health goals are just as important as genetics.

Therefore, these new channels for collaboration and communication are welcome news for beer drinkers, but this collaborative, data-rich approach has many more uses. It is especially encouraging for crops with an emphasis on quality since they frequently lack extremely large breeding organizations that can perform the high-tech equivalent of "conventional plant breeding" with their own cash. The rising democratization of high-tech plant breeding is what the case of barley demonstrates.

10.4 CANNING

The popularity of craft beer is well known. A world-class variety reflecting a wide range of styles, tastes, and origins greets customers entering any corner shop, a marked improvement from the lagers that had previously lined the same shelves for decades. However, if they pay close attention, they'll see that, more than they may expect, many of these packed craft coolers are similar to their macro-brewed forebears. A rising number of craft breweries are switching from conventional glass bottles to glossy aluminum cans. As local microbreweries grow, more and more of beers are being packaged in cans and sold in stores.

Those days when a beer can truly meant effervescent, yellow, and flavorless are long gone. Craft breweries are now canning everything from hopped-up imperial IPAs to roasty vanilla bean porters, spurred on by both industry- and consumer-driven causes.

Most can enthusiasts will concur that cans are much less vulnerable to light and oxygen contamination, cool down much faster, are easier to produce from recycled materials, and take up less space on truck beds and in shipping containers—all of which allow established craft breweries to expand their reach without drastically increasing their carbon footprint or their costs.

Cans seem to be the craft beer packaging of the future, whether they hold 10% IPAs or 3% Berliner Weisses. And, in true craft beer style, cans bring still another layer of inventiveness to the brewing process, giving brewers an appropriate platform to highlight their sometimes-underappreciated skills.

10.5 HOMEBREWING

PicoBrew of Seattle has developed contemporary, microwave-size equipment for homebrewing beer over the past five years. Aspiring brewers may take the product home and brew whatever beer they want right at their kitchen table, using homemade Pico Pak ingredient packages that are defined by breweries or by your own recipe.

And, of course, marijuana: Breweries like Corona are making investments in marijuana farms in the expectation that cannabis-infused beer may become a popular beverage in the future. Once the technology is developed and the necessary legislation is established, the goal is to produce a beverage that both beer lovers and THC fans will like.

10.6 LARGE BUSINESSES ARE DISCOVERING

After nearly two decades of witnessing the emergence of fresh, creative microbreweries, corporations like Heineken and Budweiser have not only started to imitate their methods but have also swooped in and acquired well-known firms like Seattle's Elysian Brewing to learn their trade secrets and discover fresh approaches to enter your fridge with regional flair and exotic IPA flavors.

10.7 BEER AND HEALTH

Beer is a beverage with substantial historical and cultural significance. While beer may contain certain potentially advantageous bioactive components that need additional research, interest in the possible health impacts of alcoholic drinks has mostly been on wine. The potential health advantages and dangers of low-alcohol, prebiotic, and bioactive-containing beers should be thoroughly evaluated as they are created.

Beer is one of several alcoholic beverages that have built a sizable market among health-conscious customers. Breweries have been developing various techniques to deliver healthy products to our lives. Novel brewing techniques have the potential to provide a number of health benefits, in terms of both the bioactive compounds that are derived from the ingredients and produced during the brewing process and the probiotic effects of the yeasts and other microorganisms that are in charge of the fermentation.

The challenge is to show how the bioactives—naturally occurring compounds derived from hops and fermentation, secondary metabolites produced by yeast and lactic acid bacteria—can be preserved in a product that consumers would buy without the negative effects of additional dietary calories, sugar, or alcohol.

Breweries have increased the product's nutritional value by adding vitamins, antioxidants, electrolytes, etc. Supply and demand are changing to meet these new requirements.

One of the major Spanish breweries, Estrella Galicia, is developing a beer with anti-inflammatory qualities. Chia seeds and buckwheat kasha are used to make a beer by Harpoon's Rec League. Vitamin B, minerals, and Mediterranean sea salt are also added to this beer as electrolytes.

With five beers that include potassium salts, sodium salts, and calcium salts—adding up to excellent, electrolyte-packed brews—Zelus provides one of the broadest product offerings on the market. Of course, we're referring to electrolyte-infused beers, which often have a lower alcohol content, but a non-alcoholic beer may be the healthiest choice.

10.8 LOW-ALCOHOLIC AND NON-ALCOHOLIC BEERS

It is crucial to take into account the potentially harmful effects of excessive beer intake, which are mostly related to the alcohol and energy content, together with the rising interest in the possible advantages of the substances and organisms present in beer. The hazards of excessive alcohol intake are well known, and current thinking suggests that there may not be a safe level of alcohol consumption. Moderate alcohol consumption (defined as 14 units or less per week) has been linked to a lower risk of early death and, particularly, cardiovascular disease (Holmes et al., 2016). Because of this, considerable thought should be given to new brewing methods and yeasts that could help limit or even reduce alcohol level while maximizing flavor and potential health impacts when assessing the potential advantages of beer.

Regarding the energy content, this will be taken into account once again, along with the ways the formulation and the impact of fermenting bacteria might affect the quantity of the carbohydrates, particularly residual sugar, that will be present in the finished product. Other factors to take into account are how the way the recipe is created, the brewing environment, and the fermenting bacteria affect the development of "congeners," which are chemicals connected to headache and hangover symptoms. As a result, it's critical to weigh the known harmful effects of drinking alcohol regularly, even in moderate amounts, against the possible positive effects of beer (Wood et al., 2018).

Through innovative brewing techniques frequently utilized in craft brewing, in terms of materials, brewing procedures, and types of fermentation, there is potential to increase the bioactive characteristics of beer while lowering the alcohol and energy content. Beers with lower alcohol content and more potential to enhance health may become more common as a result of consumer desire for a wider range of beer types, including alcohol-free brews. These beers may also become more popular since they are still tasty and have high consumer demand.

The market for non-alcoholic beers is likely to grow in the foreseeable future. The use of alcohol has decreased throughout Europe as a result of trends towards healthier living. Beers without alcohol are becoming more and more popular today. The non-alcoholic beer market in Poland expanded by more than 20% in 2017 (Wojcik, 2018).

Since the pandemic began, people have begun to reduce their alcohol use, largely as a result of adopting healthier lifestyles. The non-alcoholic market should expand as a result of this behavioral shift. A recent study report by Global Industry Insights projects that by 2026, this market will have generated over USD 29 billion in revenue.

Innovation still plays a crucial part. For instance, the market for global enzyme-based non-alcoholic beer is predicted to increase due to the relevance of enzymes in guaranteeing beverage quality and safety and minimizing alcohol production.

Over time, beer rose to become one of the most well-known alcoholic drinks in the world. There is a demand for a soft drink with similar organoleptic features to regular beer for many reasons, such as a healthy lifestyle, medical conditions, driving obligations, etc. There are two main ways to get such a commodity. The first step is to interfere with the biological features of beer manufacturing technology, such as altering the mashing regime, performing fermentation in ways that encourage reduced alcohol production, or utilizing unique (typically genetically modified) microorganisms. The second strategy is to make regular beer alcohol-free. This is made feasible primarily by membrane and evaporation processes.

It is necessary to establish that there is a market for such products before they can be produced. The best way to make these products using various microorganism strains may present a number of difficulties, such as varying fermenting times, higher residual carbohydrate levels because these are not used as a substrate for ethanol synthesis, or the effects of brewing to a lower alcohol by volume, which may inhibit the development of flavor. The elimination of ethanol following fermentation is an alternate strategy. Using heat to evaporate the ethanol has a tendency to produce tastes that are cooked. Heat is expected to denature possible prebiotics and polyphenols in addition to eliminating alcohol; thus, the effect may go beyond flavor (Mellor et al., 2020).

10.9 SOUR BEERS

Sour beer must be mentioned when discussing beer trends. Sour beer is created by adding bacteria to regular beer, which is fermented with a variety of brewer's yeast strains. For the production of complex flavors and tart acids, bacteria such as *Lactobacillus*, *Pediococcus*, *Acetobacter*, and others are frequently used. The unexpected contribution of bacteria, on the other hand, might take years to grow and mellow into something attractive, much like a red wine. This is in contrast to conventional brews, which are sometimes created in as little as four or five days. Sour beer, traditionally made in Belgium, has recently gained popularity among U.S. homebrewers. As a result, sour beer programs have proliferated all across the world.

Despite the fact that sour beer is very much a current trend, it's important to note that it may still be in its infancy. In the world of craft beer, the style has undeniably become "all the rage," but there is considerable disagreement about whether the craze has peaked or will continue to grow and eventually become "the new IPA," as many are dubbing it, particularly in the United States. Perhaps it won't be the new IPA. However, sour beer is a distinctive type that, if properly marketed and presented, has the potential to appeal to a very broad audience.

Sour beers, which are complex and tart and frequently taste like wine, are popular with both beer enthusiasts and non–beer drinkers. For people who don't enjoy the bitterness of most IPAs, pale ales, and lagers or the astringent roasted characteristics of porters and stouts, complex flavors and extended maturing durations with extremely low levels of hop bitterness tend to be more appealing. While it's unclear how far sour beer will go, it is undeniably a smoldering style that might very well erupt in the years to come.

Beer has a proud history and a promising future, and there are chances for the brewing sector to convince consumers of the advantages of moderate beer consumption for health and its role in a healthy lifestyle.

10.10 REFERENCES

Baker, E., Wang, B., Bellora, N., Peris, D., Hulfachor, A. B., Koshalek, J. A., Adams, M., Libkind, D., & Hittinger, C. T. (2015). The genome sequence of Saccharomyces eubayanus and the domestication of lager-brewing yeasts. *Molecular Biology and Evolution*, *32*(11), 2818–2831.

Bellon, J. R., Eglinton, J. M., Siebert, T. E., Pollnitz, A. P., Rose, L., de Barros Lopes, M., & Chambers, P. J. (2011). Newly generated interspecific wine yeast hybrids introduce flavour and aroma diversity to wines. *Applied Microbiology and Biotechnology*, *91*(3), 603–612.

Bellon, J. R., Schmid, F., Capone, D. L., Dunn, B. L., & Chambers, P. J. (2013). Introducing a new breed of wine yeast: Interspecific hybridisation between a commercial *Saccharomyces cerevisiae* wine yeast and *Saccharomyces mikatae*. *PLoS One*, *8*(4), e62053.

Bellon, J. R., Yang, F., Day, M. P., Inglis, D. L., & Chambers, P. J. (2015). Designing and creating Saccharomyces interspecific hybrids for improved, industry relevant, phenotypes. *Applied Microbiology and Biotechnology*, *99*(20), 8597–8609.

Bing, J., Han, P. J., Liu, W. Q., Wang, Q. M., & Bai, F. Y. (2014). Evidence for a far east Asian origin of lager beer yeast. *Current Biology*, *24*(10), R380–R381.

Brewer's Association. *National beer sales & production data*. Retrieved February 28, 2020, from www.brewersassociation.org/statistics-and-data/national-beer-stats/

Gibson, B., Geertman, J., Hittinger, C. T., Krogerus, K., Libkind, D., Louis, E. J., Magalhães, F., & Sampaio, J. P. (2017). New yeasts—New brews: Modern approaches to brewing yeast design and development. *FEMS Yeast Research*, *17*(4).

Holmes, J., Angus, C., Buykx, P., Ally, A., Stone, T., Meier, P., & Brennan, A. (2016). *Mortality and morbidity risks from alcohol consumption in the UK: Analyses using the Sheffield Alcohol Policy Model (v. 2.7) to inform the UK Chief Medical Officers' review of the UK lower risk drinking guidelines*. ScHARR, University of Sheffield.

Mellor, D. D., Hanna-Khalil, B., & Carson, R. (2020). A review of the potential health benefits of low alcohol and alcohol-free beer: Effects of ingredients and craft brewing processes on potentially bioactive metabolites. *Beverages*, *6*(2), 25.

Mertens, S., Steensels, J., Saels, V., De Rouck, G., Aerts, G., & Verstrepen, K. J. (2015). A large set of newly created interspecific Saccharomyces hybrids increases aromatic diversity in lager beers. *Applied and Environmental Microbiology*, *81*(23), 8202–8214.

Morales, L., & Dujon, B. (2012). Evolutionary role of interspecies hybridization and genetic exchanges in yeasts. *Microbiology and Molecular Biology Reviews*, *76*(4), 721–739.

Parker, N., James, S., Dicks, J., Bond, C., Nueno-Palop, C., White, C., & Roberts, I. N. (2015). Investigating flavour characteristics of British ale yeasts: Techniques, resources and opportunities for innovation. *Yeast*, *32*(1), 281–287.

Peris, D., Sylvester, K., Libkind, D., Goncalves, P., Sampaio, J. P., Alexander, W. G., & Hittinger, C. T. (2014). Population structure and reticulate evolution of Saccharomyces eubayanus and its lager-brewing hybrids. *Molecular Ecology*, *23*(8), 2031–2045.

Steensels, J., Snoek, T., Meersman, E., Nicolino, M. P., Voordeckers, K., & Verstrepen, K. J. (2014). Improving industrial yeast strains: Exploiting natural and artificial diversity. *FEMS Microbiology Reviews*, *38*(5), 947–995.

Steensels, J., & Verstrepen, K. J. (2014). Taming wild yeast: Potential of conventional and nonconventional yeasts in industrial fermentations. *Annual Review of Microbiology*, *68*(1), 61–80.

Wojcik, H. (2018). *Wzrasta popularność piwa bezalkoholowego: To najszybciej rosnący segment rynku w Polsce*. Retrieved May 29, 2018, from www.wiadomoscihandlowe.pl/artykuly/wzrasta-popularnosc-piwa-bezalkoholowego-to-najszy,46382

Wood, A. M., Kaptoge, S., Butterworth, A. S., Willeit, P., Warnakula, S., Bolton, T., Paige, E., Paul, D.S., Sweeting, M., Burgess, S., Bell, S., Astle, W., Stevens, D., Koulman, A., Selemer, R.M. & Thompson, S. (2018). Risk thresholds for alcohol consumption: Combined analysis of individual-participant data for 599 912 current drinkers in 83 prospective studies. *Lancet*, *391*(10129), 1513–1523.

Index

Page numbers in *italics* indicate figures or tables in the text.

C

D

E

F

R

S

T

U

V

W

Y

Z